The Faith Sector and HIV/AIDS in Botswana

The Faith Sector and HIV/AIDS in Botswana: Responses and Challenges

Edited by

Lovemore Togarasei with Sana K. Mmolai and Fidelis Nkomazana

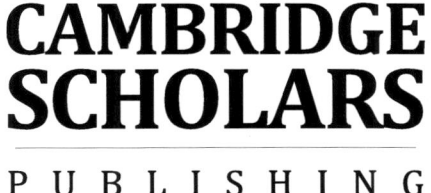

CAMBRIDGE SCHOLARS
SCHOLARS
P U B L I S H I N G

The Faith Sector and HIV/AIDS in Botswana:
Responses and Challenges,
Edited by Lovemore Togarasei with Sana K. Mmolai and Fidelis Nkomazana

This book first published 2011

Cambridge Scholars Publishing

12 Back Chapman Street, Newcastle upon Tyne, NE6 2XX, UK

British Library Cataloguing in Publication Data
A catalogue record for this book is available from the British Library

ISBN (10): 1-4438-2694-4, ISBN (13): 978-1-4438-2694-5

TABLE OF CONTENTS

List of Illustrations vii

List of Abbreviations ix

Introduction xi
Lovemore Togarasei

Part I: Background

Chapter One 2
The Botswana Religious Landscape
Fidelis Nkomazana

Chapter Two 22
"We Pray, We Give Hope": The Faith Sector Response to HIV and AIDS
in Botswana
Musa W. Dube

Chapter Three 44
The Politics of Faith-based HIV Prevention and Policies in Botswana
Kipton E. Jensen

Part II: Christianity

Chapter Four 70
 Some Mainline Churches' Involvement in Strategies to Fight HIV
and AIDS in Botswana
Sana K. Mmolai and Joseph Gaie

Chapter Five 91
Healing in the African Independent Churches in the Era of HIV and AIDS
Obed Kealotswe

Chapter Six 104
Pentecostal Churches and HIV and AIDS in Botswana
Lovemore Togarasei and Fidelis Nkomazana

Chapter Seven 117
The Use of the Bible in HIV and AIDS Contexts: Case Study of Some
Botswana Pentecostal Churches
Lovemore Togarasei

Part III: Other Religions

Chapter Eight 138
Religious NGOs and their Jihad against HIV and AIDS: The Muslim
Factor in Southern Africa
Muhammed Haron

Chapter Nine 158
The Faith of our Fathers: Collaborating with Traditional Leaders
in HIV and AIDS Response
Kipton E. Jensen and Leila Katirayi

Chapter Ten 180
Faith Based Organizations' Approaches in the Fight against HIV
and AIDS in Botswana: 1985-2009
James N. Amanze

Part IV: Religion and Culture

Chapter Eleven 208
Ntwa E Bolotse: Botswana Women, Men and HIV/AIDS
Musa W. Dube

Chapter Twelve 231
The Missing Link: Minority Languages of Botswana in the Fight
against HIV and AIDS
Joyce T. Mathangwane

Contributors 245

LIST OF ILLUSTRATIONS

Figure 1: Historical Phases of religious responses to HIV and AIDS 142

Figure 2: FBOs Responses 143

Figure 3: Select religio-ethical principles... 146

Figure 4: Muslim NGOs: their projects and programmes......................... 150

Figure 5: Google Earth Map of Mogoditshane 162

LIST OF ABBREVIATIONS

AICs	African Independent/Instituted/Initiated Churches
ARHAP	African Religious Health Assets Program
ART	Anti-retroviral Therapy
ARV	Anti-retroviral drugs
ATR	African Traditional Religion
BAIS II	Botswana AIDS Impact Survey II
BCC	Botswana Christian Council
BHP	Botswana-Harvard Partnership
BNSF	Botswana National Strategic Framework
BOCAIP	Botswana Christian AIDS Intervention Programme
BOTUSA	Botswana-United States Partnership
BTR	Botswana Traditional Religion
CBO	Community Based Organisation
CDC	Centre for Disease Control
DMSAC	District Multi-Sectoral AIDS Committee
DRM	Dutch Reformed Mission
EFB	Evangelical Fellowship of Botswana
FBO	Faith Based Organization
GDP	Gross Domestic Product
HCT	HIV and AIDS Counseling and Testing
IEC	Information, Education and Communication
LMS	London Missionary Society
MF	Ministers' Fraternal
MOH	Ministry of Health
MTP	Medium Term Plan
NAC	National AIDS Council
NACA	National AIDS Coordination Agency
NGOs	Non-governmental organizations
PEPFAR	President's Emergency Plan for AIDS Relief
PLWHA	People Living with HIV and AIDS
PMCT/ PMTCT	Prevention of Mother to Child Transmission
OAICs	Organization of African Independent Churches
OVC	Orphans and Vulnerable Children
TRS	Theology and Religious Studies
SADC	Southern Africa Development Community

List of Abbreviations

SHC	Spiritual Healing Church
SLR	Second Literature Review
STP	Short Term Plan
TB	Tuberculosis
UB	University of Botswana
UNAIDS	Joint United Nations Programme on HIV and AIDS
USA	United States of America
VCT	Voluntary Counseling and Testing
WCC	World Council of Churches
WHO	World Health Organization
ZCC	Zion Christian Church

INTRODUCTION

LOVEMORE TOGARASEI

Botswana is home to an array of religions. Over 80% of the country's people belong to one religion or the other. Religions, therefore, are better positioned to deal with HIV and AIDS. As Togarasei et al (2008:51) noted, "(religions in Botswana).....cover and extend to all segments of the population.... are well placed to influence the mass of the people at grassroots level to change their behaviour and adopt safer sex practices, ...culturally sensitive HIV prevention information and care services." The strategic position of faith organizations has been noted by many (see, for example, Parry (2003) and Chitando (2007). Even with the roll out of ARVs, faith organizations have remained strategic partners (Burchadt, Hardon and de Klerk, 2009). The government of Botswana has called for a multi-sectoral approach to HIV and AIDS response. This is in light of the devastating consequences of the pandemic in a country of less than two million people. According to UNAIDS 2010 report, in 2009 there were an estimated 300,000 adults living with HIV - or one quarter of the population aged 15 and over (UNAIDS 2010). The same report had an estimated adult HIV prevalence among 15-49 year olds of 24.8%, the second highest in the world after Swaziland. The faith sector has been a key player, positively or sometimes negatively, in HIV and AIDS response from the outbreak of the pandemic in the country in 1985. As chapter 2 of the book shall demonstrate, the government of Botswana from the outbreak of HIV and AIDS made efforts to include the faith sector in the national response. There are therefore several references to the role of FBOs in different government policies and intervention documents. Unfortunately no publication has tried to take stock of this faith sector response. This book is meant to close this lacuna.

The book covers the various religions at home in Botswana and the role they play in the struggle against HIV and AIDS. A brief history behind the production of this book is necessary for the reader. Most of the contributors in this book are members of the Department of Theology and Religious Studies of the University of Botswana. This department has taken HIV and AIDS seriously in its research strategies from the outbreak of HIV and AIDS. Rosinah Gabaitse (2008:33-46) takes stock of the various research projects that have been undertaken by members of this department individually and in teams. This book is a direct result of one of the research projects some members of the department undertook between 2006 and 2008. The project was conducted under the Ditumelo Research Project initiated by Kipton Jensen in 2005. Led by this author, the 2006 to 2008 project was commissioned by BOTUSA and funded through PEPFAR. It was meant to assess the capacity of FBOs in Botswana to prevent HIV. The results of this study are contained in Togarasei et al (2008). A number of articles in this book are based on the findings of this study.

The book is envisaged to serve both the academic and research community at national and international levels. There are now several attempts to mainstream HIV and AIDS in education both in schools and in tertiary institutions. This book therefore does not serve only those studying religion, but all who address issues of HIV and AIDS from whatever field of study.

The book comprises of twelve chapters that are divided into four parts. The first part, comprising of three chapters, provides a background of the faith sector in Botswana. In Chapter 1 Fidelis Nkomazana makes a panoramic view of the faith sector in Botswana. Looking at it from a historical perspective, he shows that various religious groups are at home in Botswana. He finds this to be partly due to the country's constitution that deliberately allows for freedom of worship and association of various religious and cultural traditions. This chapter shows the various religions that have come to operate in Botswana. The chapter provides insight into the characteristics of religion in Botswana today. It spells out the key players in the Botswana faith sector, how they came into being, how they are distributed and how they operate. Nkomazana concludes his chapter pointing out the need for such a mosaic of religions to be involved in the social, economic and political issues that affect the members of the different religions. Chapter 2 takes stock of what FBOs in Botswana have so far done in HIV response in the country. Here, Musa W. Dube first looks at the history of FBOs involvement in HIV response by revisiting government of Botswana policy documents to find out the roles assigned to FBOs. She then discusses the various activities undertaken by FBOs in areas of HIV prevention, care and support, treatment, stigma and discrimination and capacity building, as they are reflected in various national literatures. The chapter ends with an analysis of the level of success and suggestions for better FBOs involvement. The third chapter in this section, which is chapter 3 of the book, focuses on challenges that

FBOs face in responding to HIV and AIDS. Here Kipton E. Jensen explores the political circumstances that have haunted HIV prevention programs. He points out hindrances to religious collaboration such as the "identity politics" of HIV Prevention programs and policies, including "international versus Indigenous systems of knowledge and discourse of power," the politics of religious identity, both theoretically and practically, the "faith politics" of HIV prevention programs (Government Organizations and Non Governmental Organizations), as well as theoretical and practical inducements against "inter-sectoral" and "intra-sectoral" collaboration. The chapter ends with a call for all those involved in HIV and AIDS response to collaborate with each other.

Part II of the book focuses on the Christian religion and comprises of four chapters. As the first and second chapters of the book present, Botswana Christian churches are divided along denominational lines giving rise to three different categories: mainline churches, African Independent Churches and Pentecostal churches. The first three chapters address responses by three categories of churches. Chapter 4 by Sana Mmolai and Joseph Gaie discusses the response of some mainline churches to HIV and AIDS. The chapter discusses strategies employed by the selected churches to address HIV and AIDS looking at what strategies the churches consider good and bad; who approves and disapproves the different strategies and what challenges are faced in promoting the strategies. In chapter 5 Obed Kealotswe examines the healing methods and the concepts of healing in the AICs in the era of HIV and AIDS. He starts by defining the AICs with special reference to Botswana, then discusses their healing methods. Kealotswe points out healing practices that have been blamed for the spread of HIV and AIDS in Botswana before showing the changes that have taken place in the healing activities of the AICs since the outbreak of the pandemic. The chapter concludes that Botswana AICs are reversing some opportunistic infections and are now using safe methods in their practice of healing. Chapter 5, by Lovemore Togarasei and Fidelis Nkomazana, addresses the following: Pentecostal churches views of HIV and AIDS, their divine message in the light of the suffering caused by the disease, their sex education and their attitude towards condom use and issues of gender. The chapter also critiques Pentecostal doctrines and practices that hinder Pentecostal effective response to HIV and AIDS. Chapter 6 is the last one in Part II of the book. It continues discussing Pentecostal churches. In view of the centrality of the Bible in these churches, here Lovemore Togarasei focuses on how the Bible is used by the Pentecostal churches to respond to HIV and AIDS. The chapter highlights that despite the fact that the Bible was written many years ago in a completely different world from the present one, the Bible remains very influential in the lives of Christians, particularly those of Pentecostal churches. It is the first port of call particularly on questions to do with moral values and social responsibilities. Thus the Bible is used by Pentecostal churches for HIV and AIDS prevention, treatment, care and support. From an analysis of this use of the Bible, Togarasei concludes that for effective involvement of Pentecostal Christians and indeed other Christians for HIV and AIDS response, the place and function of the Bible in their lives should be taken seriously.

Part III comprises of three chapters discussing other religious groups apart from Christianity. It opens with Muhammed Haron's chapter 8 which looks at the Muslim response to HIV and AIDS. The chapter looks at the role of Muslim NGOs in their struggle against HIV and AIDS in South(ern) Africa. Haron opens his chapter by defining FBOs. He brings into view the religio-ethical principles that underpin the World Religious Systems as a whole before giving particular attention to Islam and Muslims. The chapter's second part studies the struggle undertaken by certain Southern African Muslim NGOs in fighting the pandemic. It demonstrates the extent to which these organizations have adopted a participatory approach rather than an observatory approach in dealing with HIV and AIDS. The chapter concludes that FBOs have and will continue to play a positive and dynamic role in the prevention of HIV and AIDS especially when they collaborate with the health sector. Chapter 9 presents and discusses research findings by Kipton Jensen and Leila Katirayi in African traditional healers' collaboration with the health sector. The two authors discuss traditional healers' understanding of HIV and AIDS in light of their traditional worldviews, their current contribution in collaborating with the health sector, their challenges in working with the health sector and their perception of ARVs. They conclude that traditional healers have tried to understand HIV and AIDS with its similarities to other sexual diseases and have sought to identify it with diseases they already know. Although they may lack a "comprehensive understanding of HIV and AIDS," at least from a biomedical if not also distinctively Western point of view, the chapter suggests that there is a sincere interest among Batswana traditional healers in gaining more knowledge about the virus and collaborating with biomedical practitioners. The last chapter in this part, chapter 10, is by James Amanze on some approaches that have been used by FBOs in Botswana to respond to HIV and AIDS from the outbreak of the pandemic in the country in 1985. The chapter discusses various strategies that Faith Based Organizations (FBOs) have adopted in the fight against the pandemic. It argues that the Christian churches' understanding of the nature of human sexuality has limited, to a certain extent, their choices of the means and ways of combating the scourge. Some of the strategies discussed are prayer, counseling, the establishment of day care centers, hospices, education of the masses by means of workshops, seminars and conferences and insistence on abstinence and behavior change in general. The chapter concludes that FBOs have indeed a major role to play in the prevention, care, and treatment of people living with HIV and AIDS in Botswana today.

HIV and AIDS breeds in socio-cultural and religious beliefs and practices throughout the world. Part IV of this book therefore addresses the role of culture and religion in HIV and AIDS response in Botswana. In chapter 10 Musa Dube focuses on gender inequalities. She begins by defining gender looking at what sustains it. The chapter also looks at how religion and culture construct and maintain gender. Having established this Dube then discusses how gender has become a major factor in the spread of HIV and AIDS and how it can be shot down. Chapter 12 concludes this book. In it Joyce Mathangwane argues for the need to use other indigenous languages of Botswana in the fight against HIV and AIDS. Based on selected AIDS messages from billboards, clinic notice boards and newspapers that were collected over a period of several years within the country, she observes that the use of two languages only, Setswana and English limits the effective spread of HIV and AIDS messages to Batswana. The author is of the view that even where people use a second or third language, there are certain semantic values that only a first language makes the hearer or reader relate to the message and own it personally. Mathangwane is therefore of the view that minority languages are the missing link which could allow HIV and AIDS information to effectively reach out to speakers of these languages. The chapter suggests different other social fields where these other languages could be utilised to reach out to the people, given the multi-lingual and multi-ethnic set-up of the country.

Bibliography

Burchadt, M. Hardon, A. and de Klerk, J. *Faith Matters: Religion and biomedical treatment for HIV/AIDS in Sub-Sharan Africa.* Diemen: AMD, 2009.

Chitando, E. *Living with Hope: African Churches and HIV/AIDS 1.* Geneva: WCC Publications, 2007.

Gabaitse, R. "Searching for Contextual Relevance: The Department of Theology and Religious Studies, University of Botswana's Response to HIV and AIDS," in Chitando, E. (Ed.), *Mainstreaming HIV and AIDS in Theological Education: Experiences and Explorations.* Geneva: WCC Publications, 2008.

Parry, S. *Responses of the Faith-Based Organisations to HIV/AIDS in Sub-Saharan Africa.* Geneva: World Council of Churches, 2003.

UNAIDS, *UNAIDS report on the global AIDS epidemic.* 2010.

PART I:

BACKGROUND

CHAPTER ONE

THE BOTSWANA RELIGIOUS LANDSCAPE

FIDELIS NKOMAZANA

Introduction

Various religious groups are at home in Botswana. This is partly due to the country's constitution that deliberately allows for freedom of worship and association of various religious and cultural traditions. This chapter briefly shows the various religions that have come to operate in Botswana and gives a panoramic view of the country's religious landscape. What are the characteristics of religion in Botswana today? Who are the religious players? How are the religious players distributed? How do they operate? These are some of the questions that this chapter addresses. The chapter opens by spelling out the plural character of religion in Botswana. This is followed by brief accounts of how the different religions, from ATR to new charismatic movements have come into being. The chapter concludes pointing out the need for such a mosaic of religions to be involved in the social, economic and political issues that affect the members of the different religions.

Religion and the Constitution

At independence in 1966 Botswana came with a new constitution that assisted different religions to come to the public fore and seek for ways of dialogue. The constitution of Botswana specifically stipulated and protected the rights of all citizens to have or adopt a religion of their choice. It underlined the necessity for religious freedom, expression and assembly. It also protected the right for everyone to adopt a religious belief of their choice. Individuals or groups were free to manifest their religious beliefs in worship, observance, practice or teaching as long it did not interfere with the rights of other people. Religious abuse, by restriction or discrimination by government or private actors is not tolerated. This is possibly the reason why there is no record of religious persecution or hostility to minority or unapproved religions in Botswana. This is also why there are no discriminatory legislations or policies that give preferences to favourable religions, thus disadvantaging others. Often dangerous "sects or cults" operate without stigmatization. Due to this fundamental right and policy, the indigenous religion, which dominated the life of the nation for centuries, accommodated new faiths that offered serious challenges to the extent of almost destroying it. It was always in the nature of the religion to tolerate other religions, even before the constitution made it part of the Law of Botswana. The indigenous religions of Botswana, therefore, have always welcomed other religions, and, it have, in fact, always appreciated different styles of worship, especially those similar to theirs (Amanze 2000 and Nkomazana 2001: 341-344).

Botswana has no state religion. It also prohibits forced religious instruction and participation in religious ceremonies or taking oaths that run contrary to an individual's religious beliefs. Although there are no laws against proselytizing, the proselytization that goes on cannot be termed as breaching human rights and religious freedom. From 1966, there are no reports of forced religious conversion or reports of religious prisoners or detainees or denial of migration rights on religious grounds. Although sustained interfaith committees and services have always failed, or were extremely weak before independence, the general amicable relations between the country's religious communities have always contributed to religious freedom and practice.

Botswana's policy on religious freedom can be better understood in the context of its history, culture and tradition. Although the Batswana Traditional Religion (BTR) dominated the life of the nation for centuries, it always accommodated and accepted new faiths that offered challenges in both cultural and theological terms. This was even at the extent of having the people's culture and tradition destroyed by the new religions. Very little was done to protect public safety, order, morals at the interest of fundamental rights and freedom of others.

While the constitution promotes the spirit of tolerance, it is however an expectation that all religious organizations register with the Government. To register, a group submits its constitution to the Ministry of Home Affairs. After a generally simple but bureaucratic process, the organization is registered. There are no legal benefits for registered organizations. Unregistered groups potentially are liable to penalties including fines of up to P1000 or 7 years in jail, or both. Except for the case of the Unification Church, there is no indication that any religious organization has ever been denied registration (Society Act). The practice of requiring religious groups to register before they can engage in activities such as worship is for purposes of protecting the interests, rights, safety, order and morals of the nation as a whole (Botswana Constitution, chapter 2: 3-19).

The Constitution also provides for the protection of the rights and freedoms of other persons, including the right to observe and practice any religion without the unsolicited intervention of members of any other religion. Every religious community may establish places for religious instruction at the community's expense, but prohibits forced religious instruction and participation in religious ceremonies, or taking oaths that run counter to an individual's religious beliefs. When the first Moslem members of parliament, Satar Dada, especially elected to represent the "minority groups" and Daisy Pholo, member of Parliament for Selibe Phikwe, were sworn in, they chose to use a Quran instead of a Bible. While this was the first time it happened in the history of Botswana, they were free to exercise their Constitutional right (Personal attendance, Swearing in of Parliamentarians, November, 2004).

Both government policy and the generally amicable relations among and between the country's religious communities contribute to religious freedom and practice. An independent effort to establish an interfaith committee between the Christian and Muslim communities in the early 1990's failed due to lack of identifiable mutual interests. But in matters of national interests, such as droughts and the celebration of the Botswana Day, there were efforts in the 1980s to conduct interfaith services, which only lasted for a brief period. Up to the present day, there are no reports of forced religious conversion, or refusal to allow citizen and non – citizen to return or enter the country or being forced out of the country on religious grounds. Again, there are no reports of religious prisoners or detainees in Botswana or associated with the country (Amanze, 1999).

The Constitution provides for the suspension of religious freedom in the interests of national defense, public safety, public order, public morality, or public health; however, any suspension of religious freedom by the Government must be deemed reasonably justifiable in a democratic society. When the Johane Church of God beliefs and practices seemed to deny its members and their children freedom to benefit from modern medical practice, the church met resistance from the Ministry of Health officials (Nkomazana 2009: 149). In the face of HIV and AIDS the government through the Ministry of Health has made it clear to churches like the Zion Christian Church, that they must not use healing methods that might facilitate the spread of HIV (http://www.state.gov/g/drl/rls/irf/2001/ 5573). At times, however, the state takes for granted that the churches fall under its control and seeks to bring them to its hegemony, while in actual fact, the power of the state over the churches is far more limited. On the other hand, it is evident that historic churches enjoy easy exemption, which may be an indication that the state, at times adopts an accommodating attitude on churches or religions in general. In fact, the situation of Guta RaMwari, shows that the state at times fails to confront suspected criminal acts that revolve around the notions of supernatural intervention and election, sorcery, secrecy and manipulation of humans for economic gain. Guta Ra Mwari stands as an example of an African Independent Church (AIC) which tends to inspire the majority of non members with a great deal of fear (Amanze, 1994:122-124). This is against the background of authoritarian attitude towards AICs dating back to the colonial era, when these churches were not allowed to operate. While in independent Botswana they have enjoyed more freedom, they are in comparable terms still subjected to far greater state interference, when they seek for registration with regard to their doctrine, organization and therapeutic practices, than the established churches.

With the constitution allowing freedom of worship, Botswana is now home to various religious groups. But how have the various religions come to be in Botswana. Below I briefly give an overview of the history of the various religions in Botswana.

Batswana Traditional Religion (BTR)

BTR is the oldest religion in Botswana. It is not possible to date its origins as it has always been part and parcel of the people's lives. According to John Mbiti (1975:30) "Africans are notoriously religious". This is very true of the Batswana Traditional religion which permeates every aspect of their life: ploughing, politics, funerals, crop harvest, education and even school examinations. Let us briefly look at some of the beliefs held in this religion. It is important for us to pay some attention to this religion since it influences Batswana's worldview whether they belong to it or to other religions.

Belief in a Supreme Being

The Supreme Being and Creator is known as *Modimo*. BTR constitutes the religious context in which a good number of people in Botswana live or have lived. It is believed that long before the colonial period, Batswana had a wide range of countless stories and myths explaining how the world began. *Modimo* is presented as Supreme, Creator, Source and Sustainer of life. The universe, which has its beginning in and through Him is believed to be governed and filled by Him, and without end. Their religiosity

acknowledges His reality but does not define Him.   It confesses that
Modimo is overall, unlimited and invisible. A contested aspect of indigenous
religiosity is its monotheism (Nkomazana 2005:28).

The belief in *Modimo* is not complete without the role played by
intermediaries, such as priests, kings, traditional healers, diviners,
rainmakers, family elders and most important, *badimo*, who dominate the
beliefs and practices of Batswana.   Sacrifices and prayers are offered to
them. The *badimo* are believed to be spirits of people, who lived upright
lives here on earth, died "good" and natural death at a ripe, old age and
received the acknowledged funerary rites. They could be men or women.
But male *badimo* are prominent since patriarchy is the dominant system of
the family and social integration. They are believed to be the closest link
between the physical living and the spirit world. They are also believed to
speak the language of the community with whom they lived as physical
human beings and continue to be part of their human families, who hold
them in their personal memories. In the case of a cordial relationship, they
are believed to have an interest in what happen to their families, and thus
return to visit them from time to time and symbolically sharing their
meals. They are believed to have been created by *Modimo* and to be his
subjects. People take for granted the continuation of life after death. The
relation between the living and the departed is cultivated in different ways.
This may include the use of libation (symbolic offerings), appearance of
the departed in visions or dreams of the living, naming of children after the
departed if they resemble them, and through divination. The living also
ask *badimo* to assist in conveying their prayers, sacrifices and offerings to
Modimo, since they are considered to be closer to Him than human beings.
Badimo always assume the role of mediators, intermediaries, intercessors,
and go – between *Modimo* and people.   No one can approach *Modimo*
except through the *badimo*. Belief in *badimo* is therefore an important
aspect in understanding the role of the traditional religion in Botswana. It
inculcates the ideal of harmonious living among community members
(Amanze 2000:28-70).

Family elders make regular offerings of gifts, in the form of food and
drinks to the *badimo* to reciprocate their favours. Hence, old people would
not normally eat or drink *bojalwa* (traditional beer) without first offering
some portions on the ground for them, because they are believed to be the
custodians of the land on which their children live.   They are also
guardians of community affairs, customs, traditions and ethical norms.
Offence in these matters is ultimately an offence against the *badimo*, who
act as invisible police of the families and communities. They are thought
to severely punish those who disregard the hallowed traditions of the

community, or infringe taboos and norms of acceptable behaviour in society (Amanze 2000:28-70).

Sacred Objects

Practitioners of the BTR often use sacred objects when they perform rituals. Some objects are used by individuals or families and others by the community, under the supervision of the ritual leader. Sacred objects that are considered to be very powerful are kept out of reach of ordinary people.

Communal sacred objects may be kept in the house/hut of a ritual leader, such as the rain-maker, priest or king. Much ceremony is observed when they are moved to a new place or a place where a public ritual is conducted. Ordinary people may not touch them under normal circumstances, as there are many taboos that protect them. It is believed that interfering with them brings misfortune or even death. Examples of sacred ritual objects include:

1. Divining bones called *ditaola*, used for examining and diagnosing the cause of disease, calamity or disaster that has occurred to a community, e.g. the cause of lightning that has struck a house, a person or any other object or why the rains have not come or why people are dying.
2. Drums, which are used for singing, drumming and dancing, inspire the spirit of *badimo* (ancestors) to act.

There are many other examples of such as stools used to seat a king at coronation, rain-making objects, ritual marks and dresses, herbs and charms, sacred pots reserved for ritual purposes (like those found at the Moremi sacred site), graveyards, shrines, such as those at *Lentswe – la – Baratani* in Otse and in Ramokgwebana in the North East of Botswana, which are in the form of hills and caves.

Certain animals can be regarded as sacred. The *Bakgatla*, for instance, highly respect the monkey (*kgabo*), which has now become their totem animal. When a leopard's skin is worn by a chief during coronation, it is regarded as a sign of authority and sacredness, thus treated as sacred.

Certain trees selected for ritual purposes; and beneath which sacrifices and prayers are conducted are also regarded as sacred. Such trees include the *nzeze* tree among the Kalanga of North East Botswana. The tree has great significance in the rain-making practices. There is a wide range of other sacred objects, such as strings and charms tied around the necks, arms, legs, waists of people by medical men or kept in pockets, bags, on roof tops or in other strategic places such as gates, or corners of homesteads, gates, dug in fields, kraals, etc (Nkomazana, Sacred Sites).

Sacred Literature

BTR has no sacred literature in the form of sacred scriptures or holy books. Their sacred teachings are written in the hearts, in the history and experiences of the people. All the tenets of the religion are handed on orally, sometimes with updates according to the period of time. They have religious traditions and laws governing how they worship and how they should live, which are passed from generation to generation by word of mouth. The followers of BTR are bound by the authority of their *badimo* who are believed to be very important divinities and intermediaries between *Modimo* and human beings. This knowledge or religious information is usually passed in the form of religious myths and proverbs. Some of it is associated with religious or sacred objects, and is easy to remember and pass to others, especially the young.

There are advantages with oral tradition. The lack of a written sacred literature means that there are no firm and standard doctrines and a single authority for a reference point thus allowing flexibility. One advantage, which also is a disadvantage, is that it does not have fixed sacred literature, because it provides room for flexibility. During the process of adaptation, some ideas and practices are forgotten or sometimes lost forever. The degree of sacredness of these scriptures can therefore be easily altered. The fact that most sacred scriptures were originally orally passed from one generation to another is at least also true for other religions. One of the reasons why BTR remained in this unwritten state might have resulted from the fact that its adherents were until recently an illiterate community (Nkomazana and Thompson 1998:22).

Politics, Social Justice and Religion

The pre-colonial religious institutions of the Batswana were centralized. There was a close identity and interaction between the religious and political spheres and a strong sense of common purpose between the two. The religious authorities were often the political authorities, who attempted to control reverence for royal ancestors, rainmaking, *bogwera* and *bojale* (initiation ceremonies for boys and girls respectively) ceremonies, etc. (Nkomazana 2005:26-49).

In Botswana traditional society, social justice was intended to contribute to social stability and harmonious relationships within and between ethnic groups. The expectation of the individual was largely dictated by existing religious, political and social structures, relationships, patterns and roles. The sacred and the secular were inseparable. There was no compartmentalization of life. What religion forbade or condemned, society also forbade and condemned. Society approved what religion approved and sanctioned. An offence against human beings was an offence against God and in like manner an offence against God was an offence against human beings. A code of behaviour was transmitted from generation to generation and constrained individuals to live in conformity with society.

All prohibited criminal actions and taboos such as adultery, theft, incest, unkindness to parents, lying, murder, rape, seduction, swearing falsely, were crimes and punishable. Social justice, therefore, implied conformity to these expectations. The status of women, children and men; marital laws and rules and political activities were defined by these expectations. Ritual occasions, priests, rulers, specialists, who were custodians of holy places, and ritual officers, also functioned under the same confines. Educational opportunities between the sexes were encouraged.

Both within the family and at the *Kgotla* (court or an assembly point for the discussion of communal issues), there were strict hierarchies of authority, whereby the males ruled and held responsibility for the females. Brothers ruled their sisters and sons, even their mothers, when they came to age or succeeded the inheritance. Women did not enjoy any ultimate authority or responsibility for the household. The husband was the head of the family. When women were permitted to become chiefs, it was largely a question of politico - religious symbolism; whereby a woman was treated as a man. In fact, right from childhood through adolescence and through the *bogwera* (initiation school for boys) and *bojale* (initiation school for girls), boys were trained to govern, while the training of young women concentrated on household work and the importance of submitting to the authority of men.

The traditional set–up welcomed strangers and poor people. A stranger was nearly always welcome in traditional Tswana culture because he was not an enemy. He was seen as a link with foreign parts. He brought news and information. Since his coming was a blessing he had to be shown hospitality. Whenever someone became a suspect and ran the risk of being regarded as a threat to the society as a whole, he became a social outcast. This was the worst fate to befall anyone.

The relationship between religion, social justice and order are important aspects of the traditional religions. The *Kgosi* (chief) was the central religious authority responsible for national unity, harmony and peace. He ensured that inhuman acts such as corruption, greed and theft did not exist in his society. His position was strengthened by the fact that he ruled through the *Kgotla* system, whose rules and laws were enshrined in the cultural and religious traditions of the people. As the supreme head of this institution, he was the centre of all political, social and economic activities of his town. The *Kgotla* debates promoted democratic procedures, which were characterized by political and social justice and order in their practices and conduct. It was an obligation of the *Kgotla* and the *Kgosi* to ensure that the community supported the poor, the old and strangers. After harvest some crops were kept in custody with the *Kgosi* for that purpose.

Traditional religion observed several taboos. The main purpose of these taboos as a social system was to bring social justice, order and harmony in the community. They regulated the social life and conduct of all the members of the society. Breaching the laid down laws was understood as directly offending the *badimo* and therefore creating a crisis for the rest of the community (Smith 1923:18).

Religion, social justice, morality and order are therefore inseparable in traditional Tswana beliefs and practices. They are not only believed to emanate from the *badimo*, but are to a considerable extent inherent in the social and cultural practices of the people. The people often speak of their laws as having always existed, or as having been created by God or *badimo* (Schapera 1937:197). As such the religion and cultural life of Batswana is based on sound and strong moral values. Writing about the Bakwena (a sub-tribe of Batswana), W.C. Willoughby (1928:382-3) pointed out that before the coming of Christianity the Ten Commandments were known to Batswana. He points out that reference was made to honouring the name of God, respecting parents and those in authority; punishing disobedience, cultivating self-control; hospitality, mercy and justice highly esteemed and praised; murder, stealing, adultery, witchcraft, hatred, arrogance, bearing false witness were condemned; a sense of family responsibility in meeting the social and economic needs of orphans and destitute was exercised.

In the traditional society, before the introduction of other religions, BTR provided strong moral base. It inculcated good behaviour in people. Divine wrath and punishment was believed to be a reality and the law of retribution was emphasized.

Rituals and Rites of Passage

Rites of passage are a wide range of transition rituals that mark important stages of life that are observed starting with pregnancy and at birth, initiation, engagement, marriage (wedding), procreation, status installation, and death. On the one hand the rites of passage emphasizes the role of the community, while on the other, the rites affirm the identity and importance of the individual (Nkomazana et. al 2008:40-156).

Rites of passage mark time of celebration of special events and milestones in life. They shape one's identity. They communicate meanings through participation. They take place within a religions environment. Rites are occasions for celebration and festivity marking the change of status of an individual. Rites of passage involve separation, ritual cleansing and entry to a new stage of life. Children, become adults, young women and men marry and have children, at death, the old become *badimo* and continue to assist family members.

Each rite of passage is accompanied by rituals, which are believed to be the source of protection and unity. Rituals bring order and meaning to life. It is a time when the community's collective memory is built. Religious rituals build personal and communal identity and faith. They anchor existence. Ritual experience creates, strengthens and recreates the community (Amanze 2002: 133-219).

Now that we have sketched the traditional religion of Batswana, let us consider how other religions came to be in Botswana.

The Growth of Christianity

Mainline Churches

Christianity was brought by European missionaries from South Africa. Most notable were the Scottish Congregationalist, Robert Moffat and his son-in-law, Dr David Livingstone, both agents of the London Missionary society. They were the first to preach among the Batswana. The expansion of Christianity among Batswana occurred in the 1820s when the first famous station was established at Kudumane by Robert and Mary Moffat, who headed the station for fifty years. They were joined in 1841 by the famous David Livingstone who, from there, opened up the territory to the north for missionary activity. Though also very much interested in exploration as part of missionary work, and later much more involved in the abolition of slave trade, Livingstone set up a mission station and Kolobeng amongst the Bakwena. The story of Livingstone's conversion of Kgosi Sechele I of the Bakwena is told in Livingstone's Missionary Travels (1857:chapter 1).

From Kudumane, Christianity gradually spread to the interior. Missionaries settled amongst the people, often at the invitation of the chiefs, who wanted guns and knew that the presence of missionaries encouraged the traders. By 1880 every major village or tribe in Botswana had a resident missionary and their influence had become a permanent feature of life. The missionaries worked through the chief, recognizing that the chief's conversion was the key to the rest of the tribe. The responses of chiefs varied – from Khama's (of the Bangwato) wholehearted embrace of the faith, to Sekgoma Letsholathebe's (of the Batawana) outright rejection, which he claimed was in defense of his culture. And to Sechele I (of the Bakwena) whose acceptance of Christianity created a serious dilemma for him. He did not only find himself in between his Kwena cultural beliefs and practices and Christianity, but had a tough time pleasing the missionaries on the one hand and the Bakwena on the other.

When Moffat translated the Bible into Setswana, his piety was culturally and spiritually inappropriate and uncompromising. He advised people to abandon their previous lifestyles, to fear the Christian God and hell, and to strive relentlessly towards the fruits of repentance (Dickson, 1976; Briggs and Wing, 1970).

During the last part of the 19th century, Christianity was established as the official religion of the five major Tswana states. Kwena, Ngwaketse, Ngwato, and Tawana states were served by the London Missionary Society (LMS), the Kgatla state by the Dutch Reformed Mission (DRM) and the Barolong by the Methodists.

Allegiance to the old "tribal" state churches was disrupted by incoming missions (Anglican, Seventh Day Adventist, Roman Catholic) in the early 20th century. Attendance in mission churches in general has rapidly declined since the 1950's. This particularly became evident with the coming of the more vibrant and contextual African Independent Churches and Pentecostal churches (Nkomazana 2007).

African Independent Churches

Estimating the presence of AICs among the Botswana population, Wim Van Binsbergen (http://www.shikanda.net/africa_religion/bot2a.htm), states that nearly one out of every three adults in Botswana could be counted as a member of an AIC. AICs started to flourish in the 1960s after they were brought to Botswana by migrant labourers and returning workers from South African mines and farms. Various types of these churches began to flourish among different tribes in Botswana After 1960, several new bodies began to emerge mainly as healing sects of zionist type while others were Apostolic. Although in 1966, the year Botswana gained territorial independence, AICs in Botswana only numbered some thousands, their size and influence have seen a most remarkable growth in the past centuries (Barret, 1968:24). In the 1960s there were 233 congregations of AICs with the average fewer than 800 members each out of the 262 total of registered churches in Botswana. The figure is obviously higher today.One very important factor is that Botswana state does not have a total grip on these churches. Dozens of them never registered yet functioning on a modest scale; a similar number saw their registration cancelled, yet some of these too, continue functioning outside the law (http://www.shikanda.net/africa_religion/ bot3a.htm).

The most active and popular AICs are the Zionist Christian Churches (ZCC), with headquarters in South Africa, and the Spiritual Healing Church (SHC), with headquarters in Matsiloje, ouside Francistown. These churches were particularly popular among the working class, while the Roman Catholics and the United Congregational Churches of Southern Africa (mainline churches) were popular among the middle class and the Apostolic Faith Mission and Assemblies of God (Pentecostal) were also growing fast among both working and middle classes.

There are commonly three old divisions of AICs: Ethiopians, Apostolics and Zionists. Their emergence have been explained in cultural, political and economic terms, typically associated with the impact of a capitalist economy and a colonial political environment that existed at the time.

Most of the earlier theological judgments on the AICs are largely negative. Their practices and beliefs were blamed for bringing people back to the old heathenism from which they came (Sundkler, 1961:53). Some writers referred to them as Christians, while others termed them as either syncrestic or to the extreme as non-Christians (Oosthuizen, 1979:3). The older generation of mission church officials both European and African, tended to see them as their opponets who misled their flock. The acceptance of polygamy by some of them contributed to them as being an inferior expression of Christianity or even as worse as non-Christians (Daneel, 1971:455).

Although not all AICs were political nor could their emergence be always seen as a form of direct opposition to colonialism and foreign influences generally, the origin of the fastest growing AICs in Botswana; the ZCC and SHC points to that. They engaged in activities that were regarded as "subversive" by the authorities. The SHC broke away from the Methodist church, due to its failure to incorporate Africans into the leadership role of the church and to recognize the need to contextualize its message, especially in the area of healing. The AICs contributed to African nationalism by emphasizing the idea that there was an African alternative to European values and control. They also made a significant contribution to the indigenization of Christianity and also helped people to cope with rapid change. Some like the John Masowe churches discouraged their members from visiting hospitals for medical purposes. The other factors that led to the formation of these AICs (Amanze 1994: 166-167; Nkomazana and Tabalaka 2009:137-159) are:

1. The disappointment with mainline Christianity
2. The translation of the Bible into Setswana language which opened up new possibilities to them
3. The denominational divisions and failure of the mother churches to meet local needs
4. The desire for physical healing
5. The desire for community, that is, identity, belonging and harmony
6. A response of protest against white denomination and a desire for liberation
7. A response to western cultural systems

As evident, the growth of AICs is attributed to several factors, with the factor of healing, and vibrant singing and dancing, which are uniquely African, as the most leading factors.

Pentecostal Churches

Pentecostals, who trace their denominational origins directly to the Pentecostal revival in the USA, were first introduced to Botswana via South Africa in the late 1950s and early 1960s. From the 1980s to the present there was a wave of new Pentecostal churches, some charismatic and others preferring to be classified as revivalists coming to Botswana. At the beginning of 2003 there were more than 75 registered churches falling under this category (Pentecostal) according to the Registrar of Societies, and mainly formed by immigrants from other African countries who are primarily flocking into Botswana for economic and religious reasons. This has resulted in Pentecostal churches becoming the most vibrant and fastest growing group of churches in Botswana. They are poised to become the biggest group of churches in the near future.

Pentecostal churches are however criticized for lack of adequate theology in terms of belief and practice. As such they are said to make better missionaries, than theologians, thus concentrating in writing pamphlets rather than scholarly papers and books. Most of their writings reflect personal testimony and experience than theological arguments. They emphasize healing, repentance, baptism of the Holy Spirit with evidence of speaking in tongues, and holiness, more than any other group of churches in Botswana. This, together with other factors, especially their ability to contextualize their message and practice, contributed to their rapid growth. In particular, healing, prayer and worship are the leading factors that have contributed to attracting new members to their fellowship (Nkomazana, 2009: 137-159).

Developments of Ecumenical/Umbrella Bodies: A Significant turning Point

The most important aspects of the inter and intra religious relations that took place during the period after independence was the establishment of ecumenical movements and umbrella organizations, that have played a leading role in creating forums of understanding, mutual respect and tolerance among different religions. The period after independence began to be characterized by the consciousness among Christians that the best way to solve the problems faced by the churches in the contemporary Botswana, was by working together. This involved consultations with one another and supporting one another in their mission. This awareness has been the driving force towards the formation of these organizations, with the primary objective of enhancing the spirit of ecumenism among different churches in Botswana (Nkomazana, 2007, unpublished article)

These organizations have adopted a common mission of promoting unity among the different churches in the country. The four major ecumenical organizations were founded with the aim of bringing co-operation and unity in addressing issues of national interest in the context of religion, politics and social issues. In the past, doctrinal differences contributed towards divisions and polarization of other churches. The emergence of Pentecostals and African Independent Churches, was in their early years, characterized by persecution by the mission churches. This compelled the AICs and Pentecostal churches to co-operate in order to survive. While they strongly disagreed on doctrinal issues with Pentecostal churches regarding the AICs as heretic and heathen, just like their other Western influenced counterparts in Mainline churches, they stood together during persecution.

The period from 1966 onwards therefore led to the origin and the formation of the ecumenical movement, which resulted in different denominations working together in great unity and cooperation. This gave rise to the emergence of several ecumenical and umbrella bodies, such as the Botswana Christian Council (BCC), the Evangelical Fellowship of Botswana (EFB), the Organisation of African Independent Churches

(OAICs) and the Ministers Fraternal (MF). The development of these ecumenical/umbrella bodies has also contributed to the effort of presenting the church as a united force in addressing and handling national issues (Amanze 1994 & 1997).

The University of Botswana Theology & Religious Studies department has carried out a wide range of research work in various topics on religion in Botswana. The results of these researches show that there are several important religious Christian bodies in the country. The Botswana Council of Churches (BCC) is seen as the mother organization for the ecumenical movement, for most of the historical or mainline churches and some African Independent Churches. Working very closely with the BCC is the Minister's Fraternal, a body that tries to link the government and the churches on serious issues of national interest. Pentecostal churches have their own "mother" body, the Evangelical Fellowship of Botswana, for those who are not members of the BCC. The Bible Society is also another interdenominational organization in Botswana. It affiliates more with BCC than with other ecumenical bodies. It has already translated Scriptures into Kalanga and working on the translation of the Yeyi Bible, which is in progress. The council for African Independent Churches, the Organization of African Independent Churches, is another important umbrella body. It brings together all the African Independent Churches in Botswana and the Southern African region as a whole. Scripture Union is also another interdenominational Christian organization that works in secondary schools among students throughout the country. It acts as an arm of the church in imparting Christian values to primary and secondary schools students. Flying Mission assist missionary and medical work by providing doctors, missionaries, aviation and other personnel, together with modes of transport and communication, especially to the rural areas. Other important Christian bodies that have contributed to the spiritual landscape of Botswana include the Jesus Generation Movement, which is an important interdenominational organization at post secondary level (Amanze 2006). The Joshua Project 2000, a US Evangelical Christian web site connected to Trans World Radio of Swaziland, had targeted four "unreached" ethnic groups in Botswana for conversion by the year 2000. They were the Bakalanga, the Bayeyi, the Aukwen (Auen) and the Bukakhwen (Tannekwen) in the northern part of Botswana (Neil Parsons, 1999 website).

Introduction of Other Religions to Botswana

The introduction of other religions from outside has brought interesting religious developments. The Batswana Traditional Religion/s and the missionary churches, particularly, the United Congregational Church in Southern Africa, the denomination that was formed by the London Missionary Society (LMS) missionaries, enjoyed the political support of the *Dikgosi* (chiefs) and the colonial administrators. At first, the *Dikgosi*, who were the symbols of traditional religious power, connived with the colonial and the missionaries against other religious organizations and groups (Nkomazana 1999).

Islam was introduced in Botswana by Indian traders from 1882. By 1994 it had spread to several villages, towns and cities, like Moshupa, Ramotswa, Kanye, Molepolole, Lobatse, Francistown and Gaborone. While most of its members are by and large of Indian origin, there are some Batswana and other African nationals, who have converted to the religion. Baha'i faith was introduced in Botswana in 1965; Buddhism in 1974; Hinduism in 1972 and Sikhism in 1974. The religious beliefs and practices of these religions have in many ways contributed to the creation of a multi-faith society. This has not only created an atmosphere characterized by tolerance, but also enriched the culture of the Batswana (Nkomazana, 2001:344).

Religion and Population Demography

Botswana has a total population of approximately 1,8 million. About half of the country's citizens identify themselves as Christians (Amanze, 1994). Roman Catholics, Zion Christian Church (ZCC), Spiritual Healing Church (SHC), and the United Congregational Church of Southern Africa--formerly the London Missionary Society--claim the majority of Christian adherents. There are also congregations of Lutherans, Anglicans, Methodists, the Church of Jesus Christ of Latter-Day Saints, Quakers, Seventh-Day Adventists, Jehovah's Witnesses, Baptists, the Dutch Reformed Church, and a number of independent evangelical groups, mainly the fastest growing churches of the Pentecostal and African Independent Churches type. Most other citizens (more than 50%) as mentioned above, adhere to traditional indigenous religions or to a mixture of religions. In recent years, a number of churches of West African origin were formed and draw good-sized crowds with a charismatic blend of Christianity and traditional indigenous religions. There is a small Muslim community--primarily of South Asian origin, and very small Baha'i,

Buddhist and Hindu communities -- approximately 2 to 3 percent of the population. It is unknown to have any atheists in the country.

Botswana National Atlas (2000:341) records 65% for indigenous religion and 33.95% (over 390, 0000) for Christianity. But due to the fact that majority of people mix adherence to Christianity and indigenous religions, and that there is existence of other world religions, the picture, is summarized by Amanze (1994:xi) as follows:

Christianity	392,035	(30%)
Baha'i	5, 000	(0.4%)
Muslims	3, 000	(0.2%)
Hindus	2, 000	(0.2%)
Buddhists	1, 500	(0.01%)
Sikhs	1,440	(0.01%)

With the above statistics given by Amanze, it can be estimated that the indigenous beliefs should have a population of about 69.18%. The differences in the percentages of the indigenous religion given by various scholars results from the fact that Batswana cultures are religious cultures. For them religion does not only become part of their ethos, but permeates every aspect of life, including Christianity. It is therefore not easy to estimate, the exact number of Botswana Traditional Religion (BTR) followers. Any suggested figure will always be contested as many Batswana, who belong to other religions continue to hold to some BTR beliefs and practices and therefore qualify to remain members of BTR (Haron and Jensen 2008).

As stated above, about 30 percent of the total population is Christian and about 50 percent or more hold to indigenous beliefs. Another important thing to note is that more than half of the total population is located in rural settings. When compared to twenty years ago when only 15 percent of the population lived in urban areas, this is a dramatic change. This is probably due to the fact that many people are migrating to urban centres in search of work and better standards of living. The urban population is steadily increasing due to the influence of immigrants from the rural areas. Urban centers are largely Christian, while rural ones are still predominatly indigenous in their beliefs or characterized by an indigenous type of Christianity. The type of Christianity found in rural areas is heavily influenced by the indigenous religion and culture than the type found in urban centres (Amanze 1994:xi).

Conclusion

Today Christianity is becoming the most prevalent belief system in Botswana, with possibilities of reaching over 50% of the population. Indigenous religious and medical practices, notably respect for patriarchal ancestors, have either declined or are being assimilated within popular Christian beliefs. Some of the rites of burial, wedding and birth have been adapted to Christianity and remain extremely important in Botswana life. Traditional rites of adolescent initiation for males have been retained in a few places with circumcision now being conducted in hospitals. The most important religious factor is that Botswana is increasingly becoming a multi-faith community, the spirit that is being supported in various school curricula as well as by the Vision 2016 national project.

This chapter has shown that nearly all Batswana identify with one or more of the religions at root in the country. With religion permeating all aspects of Batswana life, it is prudent upon religious groups to be found to engage not only in the spiritual lives of the adherents but also in the socio-political and economic lives.

Bibliography

Amanze, J. "Religious Pluralism in Africa: Some notes on the interaction between African traditional religions, Christianity and Islam in the 19th and 20th centuries", *Scriptura: International Journal of Bible, Religion and Theology in Southern Africa*", Vol.74:3, 2000, 325-340.

—. *A History of the Ecumenical Movement in Africa*. Gaborone: Pula Press, 1999.

—. *Botswana Handbook of Churches, Ecumenical Organizations, Theological Institutions and other World Religions*. Gaborone: Pula Press, 1994.

—. *Ecumenism in Botswana: The Story of the Botswana Christian Council*. Gaborone: Pula Press, 2006.

—. *African Traditional Religions and Culture in Botswana*, Gaborone: Pula Press, 2002.

Barrett, D. B., *Schism and Renewal in Africa: An Analysis of Six Thousand Contemporary Religious Movements*. Nairobi: Oxford University Press, 1968, reprint 1970.

Briggs and Wing, *The Harvest and the Hope*. Johannesburg: UCCSA, 1970.

Daneel, M.L., "Shona Independent Churches & Ancestor Worship", in
Barrett, D.B. (ed.), *African Initiatives in Religion*. Nairobi: East
African Publishing House, 1971.

Dickson, K. *The Human Dimension in the Theological Quest*, Accra:
Ghana Universities Press, 1976.

Gulbrandsen, O. "Missionaries and Northern Tswana rulers: Who used
whom?" *Journal of Religion in Africa*, 23:1, 1993, 44.

Haron, M. and Jensen, K. E. "Religion, identity and public health in
Botswana," *African Identities*, Vol. 6:2, 2008, 183 – 198.

Livingstone, D. *Missionary Travels and Researches in South Africa*. New
York: Harper and Brothers, 1868, 1st edition 1857.

Maphanyane, J. and Mokopakgosi, B. "Democracy, Government and
Politics", *Botswana National Atlas*. Gaborone: Department of Surveys
& Mapping, 2001, 345-356.

Mbiti, J. *Introduction to African Traditional Religion*, London:
Heinemann Educational, 1975.

Nkomazana, F., etal, *Religious & Moral Education for Everyone:
Learner's Book Standard 7*. Gaborone: Macmillan, 2008.

Nkomazana, F. and Tabalaka, A. "Aspects of Healing Practices Methods
among Pentecostals in Botswana – Part 1" *Boleswa Journal of
Theology, Religion & Philosophy (BJTRP)*, Vol. 2:3, 2009, 137-159.

Nkomazana, F "Some evidence of belief in the One True God Among the
Batswana before the missionaries", in *BOLESWA Journal of Theology,
Religion and Philosophy*, Vol. 1:1, 2005, 26-49.

—. "Sacred Sites in Botswana", Ongoing and unpublished research,
Department of Theology and Religious Studies, University of
Botswana.

—. Ongoing research on Pentecostalism, Department of Theology &
Religious Studies, University of Botswana.

—. "The First Missionary Encounter Among the Batswana: A Case study
of the Bangwato of Shoshong, 1857-1871," Nkomazana, F. and
Lanner, L. (eds.), *Aspects of the History of the Church in Botswana*.
Pietermaritzburg: Cluster Publications, 2007, 50-209.

—. "The Story of King Sechele 1 and the Missionaries," *Journal of
Religion and Theology in Namibia*, Vol.2, 2000, 95-109.

—. "London Missionary Society, Church and State in a Colonial
Bechuanaland: The Case of Bangwato, 1857-1923," *Scriptura:
International Journal of Bible, Religion and Theology in Southern
Africa"*, Vol.71, 1999, 303-312.

—. "Livingstone's ideas of Christianity, Commerce & Civilization," *Pula:
Botswana Journal of African Studies*, Vol. 1 & 2, 1998, 44-57.

—. "Rural Churches in Churches: A Case of Jakalasi 2 Village", in *Scriptura International Journal of Bible, Religion and Theology in Southern Africa"*, Vol. 93, 2007, 352-369.

—. "Faith Healing as a Challenge to Religion in Botswana" A Paper presented at the BOLESWA Conference, University of Swaziland, 2002.

—. Development of Ecumenical/Umbrella Bodies in Botswana, unpublished paper, 2007.

Oosthuizen, G. C. *Theological Battleground in Asia & Africa: The Issues Facing the Churches and the Effects to Overcome Western Divisions.* London: C. Hurst & Company, 1972.

Sales, J. M. *Planting of the Churches in South Africa.* Michigan: William B. Eermans, 1971.

Schapera, I. *The Bantu Speaking Tribes of South Africa.* London: Routledge & Kegan Paul, 1937.

Smith, E.W. *The Religion of Lower Races: as illustrated by the African Bantu.* New York: Macmillan, 1923.

Sundkler, G. *Bantu Prophets in South South Africa*, London: Oxford Press, 1961.

Willoughby, W.C. *The Soul of the Bantu*, London: SCM, 1928.

http://www.shikanda.net/african_religion/Bots3.htm

http://www.state.gov/g/drl/rls/irf/2001/5573

CHAPTER TWO

"WE PRAY, WE GIVE HOPE":
THE FAITH SECTOR RESPONSE TO HIV
AND AIDS IN BOTSWANA

MUSA W. DUBE

Introduction: Botswana's Religious Mosaic
and HIV and AIDS Response

Botswana is a multi-religious society which espouses freedom of religious
affiliation and worship in its constitution. Thus *Vision 2016: The Long
term Vision for Botswana* (1996:12) states that, "no citizen of future of
Botswana will be disadvantaged as a result of gender, age, religion or
creed, color, national or ethnic origin, location, language or political
opinions." As chapter one of this book has shown, active religions in
Botswana are African Indigenous Religion, Christianity, Islam, Baha'i
Faith, Hinduism and Buddhism. While the rest of faiths are organized
religions that often require one to be either born and raised in the faith or
to make an individual choice, in African Indigenous Religion one is born
into the culture and need not make any choice, proclamation, conversion
or to read and follow a particular scripture, rather to be born in an African
community and to live by the values of its culture. In African Indigenous
religions there is no separation of the scared and the secular. Consequently;

> It should be pointed out from the outset that it (is) was difficult to identify
> the followers of African Traditional Religion in Botswana. This is
> because…whilst many Batswana embraced Christianity, they still needed a
> religion defined on the basis of their traditional rituals. This being so, many
> Batswana find themselves in two worlds (Togarasei et. al. 2008: 26).

Many of those who have accepted some other religions still find
themselves practicing some form of traditional religion. As a result,

although all Africans can be said to belong to ATR in Botswana (Togarasei et al 2008:15), only the two traditional healers' associations, Botswana Dingaka Association and Dingaka tsa Setso Association remain the custodians of the religion.

The majority of Batswana claim to be Christians. There are therefore many Christian churches. These are often divided into three major categories: Mainline/Mission Churches, African Independent Churches and Pentecostal/Evangelical Churches. Apart from the individual Christian churches, Christianity also has umbrella organizations that are groupings of the individual churches. These are the Botswana Christian Council (BCC), consisting mainly of mainline churches; Evangelical Fellowship of Botswana (EFB), consisting mainly of Pentecostal/Evangelical churches and Organization of African Instituted Churches (OAICs), consisting of African Independent Churches. Not all individual churches, however, belong to these umbrella groups. As this paper highlights, these three national ecumenical organizations in Botswana have declared an all out war against HIV and AIDS.

The term 'faith-based organisations' is often used to describe religions and religious groups. But although the term "faith-based organizations" (henceforth FBOs) has been used internationally, it does not have a universally accepted definition. Most Botswana HIV and AIDS strategic documents assign specific roles to Faith Based Organizations, without defining their identity. Togarasei et al (2008:15) define an FBO as, "a group of people sharing the same location (by often meeting regularly at some place), similar spiritual beliefs, shared communal goals and social responsibilities." In other sources FBO refers to any charity or non-profit organisation aligned to any one of the world's major religions (www.wikpedia.org/wiki/faith-based). A common denominator of these citations is that FBOs are linked to religion(s). In this chapter, I follow Togarasei (2009) and treat as FBOs all religious groups, their associations, umbrella groups and charitable organizations founded by faith communities. Thus to understand FBOs in Botswana one has to take cognizance of the multi-religious landscape of the country described above.

From the outbreak of the HIV epidemic in 1985, Botswana has demonstrated a strong and committed response characterized by a series of strategic plans. The first response was a short term plan (STP) that focused on HIV and AIDS diagnosis and production of Information, Education and Communication (IEC) material. Thereafter, the country embarked on a multi-sectoral response to HIV and AIDS that included both the health and non-health sectors-based HIV and AIDS interventions. The programmes were implemented in Medium Term Plan *(MTP) 1*(1989-1993), *MTP 2*

(1997-2002), *Botswana National Strategic Framework* (BNSF) (2003-2009), *National Strategy for Behaviour Change Interventions and Communication for HIV and AIDS* (2006-2009), *National Operational Plan for Scaling Up HIV Prevention in Botswana* (2008-2010) and the *National Campaign Plan: Multiple Concurrent Partnerships* (2009). There have also been other strategies for specific-sectors or population groups and areas. Some good examples here included the *Action Plan for People with Disability and HIV/AIDS in Botswana* (2005-2007), *Botswana Safe Male Circumcision: Add-on Strategy for HIV Prevention* (2008) and *FBOs Strategy on HIV Prevention, Treatment and Care and Support (2009-2016).*

The Botswana national HIV and AIDS instruments consistently feature FBOs, with their role increasingly being better and wider with time (NACA 2006:15). For example, *MTP II: (1997-2002)* points out that, "There is now better cooperation and support by most religious organizations" (1997:27). In the *BNSF*, FBOs are featured frequently under the operationalisation of district responses (2003:37-55). The *National Strategy for Behavior Change Interventions and Communications for HIV and AIDS* also lists FBOs as one of the actors in the structures of national response to HIV and AIDS (2006: 1, 15, 17 & 27). *Oicheke, National Campaign Plan: Multiple Concurrent Partnership,* launched in March 2009, also greatly features FBOs in its development stage, listing a number of participating FBOs such as BOCAIP, Ministers Fraternal, Evangelical Fellowship of Botswana, Botswana Christian Council, Love Botswana, True Love Waits, Ghanzi Christian AIDS Committee.

Consequently, in this chapter, I seek to sketch the FBOs response and its link to the national response in the past twenty-eight years. This will be attended under the following subheadings: Botswana's FBOs and Health, Prevention, Care and Support, Treatment, Stigma and Discrimination and Capacity Building

Botswana's FBOs and Health

Historically religions have always been involved in health matters. In African Indigenous Religions, health was the realm of *Dingaka tsa setso* (traditional healers), whose approach to health capitalized on healing of relationships, using rituals and herbs (Dube 2001:179-198). The arrival of Christianity during colonial times was accompanied by two strategies of evangelism: the school and the hospital (Amadiume 1987). Indeed Africa wide churches allegedly still provide up to 60% medical services (ARHAP 2006). In Botswana this is exemplified by the Lutheran founded hospital in Ramotswa; Seventh-Day Adventist founded hospital in Kanye; and Dutch Reformed founded hospital in Mochudi, which preceded government health facilities.

FBOs health assets and services, however, are much wider than medical services in the form of hospitals or curing the body. Rather religious health assets are holistic and include creating healing and healed communities, through promotion of moral individuals and communities, giving hope and promoting faith (Cochrane and Schimd 2004:6). In the HIV and AIDS era, it has been even more evident that health is achieved when the society embraces healthy relations at family and community levels. FBOs are unparalleled in promoting healthy communities and individuals through the promotion of the fear of God, respect of the other, respect of the self, respect of the community and environment and being compassionate to the suffering. In this basket of wellbeing, health includes physical, mental, spiritual and social well-being. In the HIV and AIDS era, these non-medical FBOs health assets make religions more central for promotion of social justice, abstinence, faithfulness, care for orphans, care and support for PLWHA, advocacy for access to affordable treatment, promotion of compassion instead of stigma and discrimination and accompanying the sick and the bereaved. For example, the ethics of *Botho* (Gaie and Mmolai 2007) in African Indigenous Religion of Botswana has been a tremendous force in that they encouraged Botswana communities and families to absorb orphaned children and to care for sick relatives, when the hospitals could no longer cope with HIV and AIDS. Consequently, FBOs have been inevitably involved in the past 28 years of living with HIV and AIDS in Botswana and the world, as attested by the national strategic plans (MTP II 1997-2002:28-51 BNSF 2003:43-55). According to *Botswana National Strategic Framework for HIV/AIDS 2003-2009,* Faith-Based Organizations:

- Provide community leadership and guidance
- Mobilize resources for HIV/AIDS interventions
- Undertake advocacy initiatives
- Provide counseling, care and support to orphans and PLWHAs
- Work closely with DMSACs
- Provide abstinence amongst the youth and delaying sexual debut (2003: 71)

This chapter thus seeks to highlight some FBOs best practices, which will inform the future FBOs response to HIV and AIDS. I must point out in advance that while literature indicates that Botswana FBOs are quite committed to the HIV and AIDS, however, it is primarily the Christian and African Indigenous Religions *dingaka* that are largely involved. Other religions such as Islam, Baha'i, Buddhism and Hinduism are hardly visible. This does not mean they are not doing anything (MOH 2009), but obviously their minority numbers may not allow comprehensive involvement. While they may not have the same number of followers as in Christianity and African Indigenous Religions, they need to find their strength, such as financial resources and other ways of contributing to the national HIV response. This may involve such strategies as collaboration with other FBOs, advocacy, regular compassionate activities, and volunteering in particular projects. This chapter seeks to map out FBOs activities in the following areas: prevention, care and support, treatment, stigma and discrimination and capacity building, as they are reflected in various national literatures.

Prevention

Botswana Christian AIDS Intervention Programme (BOCAIP) is the longest, and by far the most countrywide reaching HIV and AIDS FBO. BOCAIP was formed in 1999 by churches and other para-church organisations in response to the then President Sir Ketumile Masire's 1996 declaration of the month of September as a month of prayer for the country and its people because of HIV and AIDS (BOCAIP, undated). According to *Botswana National Strategic Framework for HIV/AIDS 2003-2009,* "church communities make up this organization (BOCAIP) which aims to prevent the spread of HIV/AIDS through community education and outreach programmes" (2003:70). BOCAIP runs several prevention projects. Peer Mother Project, focusing on PMCT, is described below under treatment. "Prevention through Behaviour Change is a project on two sites, Masunga and Kanye. Its objectives are to "promote abstinence among youth aged 10-17; promote parent-child communication in areas of HIV/AIDS/STIs and sexuality." BOCAIP also runs a Youth Voluntary Counselling and Testing (VCT) centre, based in Ramotswa, which focuses on youth aged 16-25. Its objectives include, "to increase demand to HIV testing among youth and to contribute to reduction of HIV incidence among youth." Recently they opened up three youth VCT projects in Maun, Francistown and Molepolole. The theme of this testing project is "Making HIV testing a priority" (BOCAIP, Newsletter, April 2009). According to the BOCAIP Newsletter;

In each site there are selected peer educators. Their role is to mobilise the community, promoting VCT among youth and disseminating information on important issues to young people. Peer educators work hand in hand with trained counsellors who offer counselling and testing services.

The Evangelical Fellowship of Botswana (EFB), a grouping of evangelical and Pentecostal churches, also runs HIV and AIDS projects. In his worship notes at the Faith Based HIV/AIDS Summit 1-5th December, 2003, Pastor Dan Joshua Yang of the EFB held that, "life is sacred, important, dedicated and special because it is designed to give us the experience of God and daily....," (2005: 18). Speaking to the churches about HIV prevention he underlined that "God wants us to protect the vessel by taking care of it, preserving and protecting" (18). Accordingly, the 2008 EFB annual report notes that:

> The two and half years of the pilot project have been an exciting period. The Project initially was to focus on HIV/AIDS prevention, counselling, Orphan care and Home based care, but due to donors' interest in prevention, EFB pilot project for the last two years has focused on HIV/AIDS prevention. The project objectives and implementation plans for the last two years have been successfully implemented (Munamunungu 2008:27).

FBOs claim to have been largely associated with abstinence when it comes to HIV and AIDS prevention. However, data on the ground suggests otherwise. For example, Botswana Christian Council ran a national project on Adolescents Sexual Health, which has since ended due to lack of donor funds. In one of its earliest surveys, run by Kgolagano College in 2003 (it has been hard to find the final report of the project) they report that when churches are assessed individually or by families, there is greater tolerance towards other methods of prevention than just abstinence, as often assumed. The findings indicate that when it comes to abstinence only as a method of prevention, 28.5% embrace it among African Independent Churches (AICs); 73.6% among evangelicals and 55% among the mainline churches. When it comes to abstinence and condom use as methods of prevention, then AICs account for 21.4% ; the Evangelicals for 21% and the mainline churches for a mere 8.3% (BCC 2003: 7).

The recently completed countrywide *Assessment of the Capacity of Faith-Based Organizations for HIV Prevention in Botswana* (Togarasei et. al. 2008:8) lists the following as key FBOs' prevention activities:

- " Preaching or otherwise teaching abstinence and fidelity
- Encouraging condom use both among the married and unmarried. They however, hold different opinions when it comes to condom use by the unmarried.
- Providing counseling services
- Empowering youth with risk avoidance life skills, sometimes in the form of abstinence clubs
- Prayer
- Encouraging HIV testing
- Discouraging stigmatization"

The study also points out that FBOs are confronted with a number of challenges in implementing their HIV prevention programs. These include:

- "Inadequate financial resources (67%)
- Inadequate facilities (54%)
- Inadequate technical skills and training among members (49%)
- Insufficient staff to implement HIV prevention program (47%)" (Togarasei et. al. 2008:9).

These findings are consistent with some of the above described findings from various FBOs bodies.

National HIV and AIDS instruments consistently feature FBOs, with their role increasingly becoming better and wider with time. *MTP II* (1997-2002) notes that:

> ...some religious organizations were initially reluctant to accept some aspects of HIV interventions such as condom promotion and inclusion of HIV prevention in Family Life Education (FLE). However, with increased awareness and better understanding of the epidemic, the situation has changed. There is now better cooperation and support by most religious organizations. Several religious organizations are actively involved in addressing the HIV epidemic through a variety of targeted prevention ... activities (27).

In the *MPT II* strategy, under institutional strengthening, "support for religious NGOs and CBOs providing moral education activities for adolescents" (51) is advocated and under service delivery, strengthening "the provision of moral education to influence the delay of early sex initiation," (51) is also encouraged.

In the BNSF (2003-2009), FBOs are featured more frequently under the operationalisation of district response (37-55). Several districts mention FBOs for prevention activities some of which reads: "Increase age of first sex by promoting abstinence and virginity through primary schools and churches" (43); "Develop and disseminate prevention and related behavioral change communication (BCC) aimed at the vulnerable groups, especially the youth, using media and churches;" (44); "…mobilize churches and schools to promote abstinence, avoidance of premarital sex among youth, and faithfulness among married couples" (46); "Orient traditional healers on HIV/AIDS prevention e.g. sterilization of instruments" (47). Most importantly, the role of FBOs in the implementation of national strategies for HIV prevention is that FBOs are actively involved in various activities mentioned by the BNSF, such as behavior change and promotion of VCT. Accordingly, the introduction to the *National Strategy for Behavior Change Interventions and Communications for HIV and AIDS* lists FBOs as one of the actors in the structures of national response to HIV and AIDS (2006:1). However, *Behaviour Change Interventions and Communication Strategy for the Health Sectors* scantily features FBOs (2006:22, 23, 32), which is underutilization of FBOs skills and interest on behavior change. For example, the *Progress Report of the National Response to the UNGASS Declaration of Commitment on HIV/AIDS* has listed some of FBOs behavior-change programs among best practices (2008:30). Similarly, the *National Operational Plan for Scaling Up HIV Prevention in Botswana (2008-2010)* acknowledges that, "VCT is provided mainly by NGOs such as Tebelopele and BOCAIP" (2008:11) and that, "Political, religious and community leadership, reinforced by supportive media coverage, can portray multiple partnerships as a threat to individual and public health" (40).

In a recent Ministry of Health (MOH) rapid assessment of FBO activities, prevention gets the highest passion among FBOs of Botswana.

Most FBOs emphasize abstinence in their preaching. Common responses to what their organizations were doing for HIV prevention were "preach abstinence to the single," "preach abstinence and faithfulness," and "preach abstinence to the youth." FBOs are generally agreed that the only way to turn the tide of HIV is to teach all those who are not married to abstain. This message is supported by their sacred literature (scripture) and Botswana traditional beliefs and practices. Sex, which is the major source of HIV infection, they teach, should only be practiced in the marriage institution.   While preaching abstinence cuts across all FBOs, it is emphasized among Pentecostal and mainline churches, particularly those in the urban areas. To promote abstinence by the youth, some FBOs especially those from the main line churches in urban areas have established Abstinence Clubs for their youths and unmarried. One FBO (BA/GB) said they teach moral development for children, both those from their faith and those from other faiths (2009: 25).

In the 2003 Faith-Based HIV/AIDS Summit of 1st-5th December, K. Ampomah of the UNAIDS noted that:

> In the past, the church has been involved mainly in care and support for HIV/AIDS patients. Prevention was only advocated for in traditional ways where the church demands abstinence for the unmarried and faithfulness for the married. Whereas these efforts are commendable they are not sufficient as seen by increased teenage pregnancies in the church. The church needs to teach youth sexuality and repackage the existing prevention messages so that they have more impact (2005:41).

Clearly the FBOs commitment to prevention remains largely focused on teaching and preaching about abstinence and faithfulness. The limitations noted by Ampomah back in 2003 are openly acknowledged by the FBOs in 2009, who state that they need to diversify their methods of teaching and to make them appealing to young people in particular and to enhance faithfulness by embarking on marriage enrichment (MOH 2009:54). FBOs also need to grasp the structural issues such as poverty and gender inequalities that make abstinence and faithfulness less successful, hence to be more open towards risk reduction methods (condom use, delayed sexual debut), rather than insisting solely on risk avoidance (abstinence, faithfulness).

Care and Support

According to Ezra Chitando;

> As a healing community, the church offers love and friendship. It offers a shoulder to cry on for the bereaved. It visits the sick and the lonely. It cares for grandmothers and children who provide care to orphans. It pays fees for the education of orphans. It listens to the abused women and children. It takes up the rights of those of us with HIV or AIDS. As a healing community, the church binds wounds and heals memories. It is 'a church of all and for all' (2007: 73).

Turning to some of the care and support case studies in Botswana, BOCAIP runs Orphan Care (orphans and vulnerable children) and HIV and AIDS Counseling and Testing (HCT). The objective of the latter is "to increase access to counseling and testing services." Its activities include on-site HCT, provision of post test education and to undertake community outreach." BOCAIP's Care for OVC project covers six sites around the country and has approximately 1544 OVCs registered in its centers. The activities of the project include "Day care, Kid camps, Caregiver support, child counseling and psycho-social support materials." As the above quote from Evangelical Fellowship report indicates, their activities also include, "counselling, Orphan care and Home based care" (Munamunungu 2008:27).

Turning to individual churches, Anglican and Roman Catholic Churches have been on the forefront of care and support. The Roman Catholic Church has been running Pre-school and Day-Care centres for orphaned children, an Orphan school in Mogoditshane and a home-based Care program for working members of families who have sick people in Mogoditshane, Metsimotlhabe and Mmopane (Nkomazana 2007:56). The Anglicans Communion runs a pre-school and day care centre for orphaned children and a Hospice for working families with sick members (56).

MTP II (1997-2002) notes that "several religious organizations are actively involved in addressing the HIV epidemic through... home based-care activities and hospice and AIDS care" (1997: 28). In the BNSF (2003-2009) several districts mention FBOs for care and support activities some of which read: "strengthen referral mechanisms between traditional healers, faith-healers and health systems in order to improve utilization of treatment and care services" (2003: 40); "facilitate support services for People Living With HIV and AIDS (PLWHAs) across the district, like FBOs for emotional and spiritual support" (54); "support existing church programmes to increase outreach to the infected and affected" (56); while BOCAIP is also noted for running programs that seek to "mitigate the impact of HIV and AIDS on individuals and communities through counseling and orphan care" (70).

The contribution of FBOs to the national response to HIV and AIDS is, however, measured by the extent to which they have actively undertaken several activities mentioned in the BNSF such as strengthening home-based care, orphan care programs, opening day care centers, training more counselors, promoting PMCT and providing care to mobile populations (immigrants). Indeed, the *Progress Report of the National Response to the UNGASS Declaration of Commitment on HIV/AIDS* has recognized some of FBOs psycho-social services to youth as best practices (2008:34). Be that as it may, the recently published *National Situation Analysis on Orphans and Vulnerable Children in Botswana* points out that the government is the major provider in OVC services, while NGOs, CBOs and FBOs are small players (2008: 79). The report holds that "NGO/FBO/ CBOS are providing psycho-social support but they have limited coverage due to lack of counseling skills" (108). The report thus recommends that it is necessary to "explore avenues of enhancing the capacity of NGOs, CBOs and FBOs in contributing to OVC support" (139).

The MOH 2009 rapid assessment of FBOs response to HIV and AIDS highlights that FBOs are actively involved in HIV and AIDS care and support. The report found the following FBOs' care and support services:

> Methods used include psycho-social support (counseling, giving hope and praying for PLWHA, orphans and the affected); giving physical care to the sick by visiting the sick in their homes and joining home-based care programs; providing material needs such as food, accommodation, clothes and transport; encouraging testing, adherence to ARVs and providing education for pre-school orphans. Building/renting and running facilities for counseling, hospices and day-care centers for orphans and vulnerable children (MOH 2009: 57).

In the light of these findings, the report recommended that:

> ...these methods need to be continued, strengthened and expanded to reach more places and people countrywide and to be more qualitative. This should involve encouraging and empowering more FBOs to be involved in care and support of orphans and PLWHA either through collaborating with existing programs (with other FBOs, stakeholders and government) or beginning new care and support programs (many did not have any project) countrywide (57).

Treatment

In her paper, "Rebuilding Botswana: The Gospel and the Challenge of HIV/AIDS," presented at the Botswana Faith-Based Summit 1-5th December 2003, Dube sought to build a theological foundation for care, support and treatment. Reading from Luke 4: 16-22, she held that,

> In all the four gospels there is an overwhelming attestation that apart from teaching, Christ spent a better part of his earthly ministry healing the sick....It is important that the church must realize that Christ healed physical bodies of those who are sick, but he also healed the mind, the spirit and their social health. Indeed these are inseparable (2005: 56).

Available literature is largely silent on Botswana FBOs' involvement in treatment. Since ART has been primarily run by hospitals, FBOs have not yet embarked on massive programs in the area. Be that as it may, the national outcry about some church leaders who encourage people on ART not to adhere, thus running the risk of developing multi-drug resistant TB and HIV, has been widely published in the papers (The Botswana Guardian, 25 May 2007). This in itself points to the need for more education and involvement of FBOs in the promotion of adherence to treatment.

One good model is the BOCAIP's Peer Mother Project, which has been running since 2005 in 14 sites of the country. Its objectives are to "promote male involvement in PMTCT and increase partner testing; increase baby testing; promote networking relationships with health facilities; empower the community through the training of HIV+ women and partners with PMTCT information; mobilize family members and community to support PMTCT."

As part of treatment, some FBOs are involved in the provision of ARVs. Togarasei et al (2008:37) mention one Roman Catholic Church parish in Francistown that provides free ARVs to those people who cannot access government support, particularly the immigrants. In the BNSF the provision of treatment is placed together with care and support, which is reviewed above. Concerning the role of FBOs, BNSF seems to associate them with referral. For example, traditional healers are listed as partners in the "development of referral systems" (2003:33); and the need to "strengthen links between traditional healers, FBOs, NGOs and DMSAC in order to increase utilization of care, treatment and support services" (52) is acknowledged.

In the MOH 2009 rapid assessment of FBO's HIV and AIDS activities, FBOs underlined that they do not treat, rather they pray and give hope to people and then refer them to medical health facilities. "We pray; we give hope," was a constant refrain among FBOs, when it came to treatment. Giving hope included encouraging people to seek health care facilities and encouraging people to adhere to ARVs. Praying for them means praying for the ARVs to work positively in the body of a client. There was no attestation of FBOs who discouraged people from adhering to their medication. The trend was collaboration with the health sector in the provision of holistic health. However, FBOs, have not completely handed over physical health to the medical sector. The Roman Catholic Church continues to provide ARVs to groups that have no access to government health services, while other mainline churches have also expressed interest in providing the same medical services. Moreover, FBOs have not surrendered the search for HIV cure to the medical sector. African Indigenous Religions and the African Indigenous Churches, in particular,

are also searching for HIV and AIDS cure. While the latter continue to
refer clients to the medical guild and encourage adherence to ARVs, they
are also using their own treatment as immunity boosters and quite
disappointed that so far they have not cracked the nut of finding the HIV
cure (MOH 2009:38). In short, FBOs have not surrendered their historical
role for physical healing to the health care facilities, but consider
themselves as partners in holistic health. The findings of the MOH rapid
assessment on treatment is best captured by the following quote:

> Most FBOs regard all healing as God's will for all the sick regardless of
> whether it is delivered through medicine/herbs or faith. Consequently,
> FBOs pioneered the provision of medical services not only in Botswana
> and Africa, but also worldwide. Accordingly data indicates that almost all
> FBOs have a twin approach to AIDS treatment; namely, providing spiritual
> support to people (giving hope to the sick, praying for the sick, counseling)
> while at the same time referring PLWHA to health services (for testing,
> beginning ART and adherence) (2009:57).

Unfortunately, there is no indication that the medical health sector is
willing to treat FBOs as equal partners in provision of holistic health.
Consequently, it is encouraged that FBOs should refer clients to the
medical health sector and encourage those on ARVs to adhere to their
treatment as a one way street. The medical health sector (which is actually
a western-based medicine) is not expected to refer some of their clients to
FBOs for health services. The practice is what it is—a colonial
framework, which regards all that is western as best and the standard, so
much so that the medical practices that sustained our communities for
centuries are now relegated to the boxes of baseless superstition. Even so,
the memories of the medical health sector here are so short—forgetting
that just about every western medical hospital in Botswana was first
introduced and run by the church. FBOs are not strangers to all forms of
medical and health practices and services. Be that as it may, the
emergence of some fly by night Pentecostal preachers, who have seen
ARVs and God's power as fighting competitors in a boxing ring, by
insisting that once they pray for clients on medications, the latter must
abandon their medication has been troubling. Gladly, these preachers are
not representative, or even in the minority, but some aliens that land and
go. They do, however, highlight that it is important to underline that there
is no conflict between prayer and being on medication, for all good gifts
come from God. It is therefore unnecessary for some FBOs to put God
and ARVs in a competition to suppress HIV. A theology of peaceful
existence of God and the ARV will be in order, for the implications for

divergence will be too costly to entertain. As Ezra Chitando underlines, "There is an urgent need to develop an African theology of healing in contexts of HIV and AIDS. Such a theology should synthesize the different therapeutic systems operating in most African countries: traditional healing, Christian faith healing and biomedicine" (2007:70).

Stigma and Discrimination

In the beginning, FBOs were notoriously marked for promoting stigma by equating HIV and AIDS with sin and God's curse (Chitando 2007:19-26; Dube 2008:145-167). Recalling this humbling history among churches, Chitando points out that:

> The Bible was read in ways that condemned people living with HIV. The issue was simplistically reduced to one of individual or personal morality. Vulnerability to infection was understood solely in terms of whether or not one was sexually promiscuous. People living with HIV were regarded as individuals who did not live up to the high moral standards (2007:19).

This unfortunate stance was partly a result of ignorance and the newness of the disease and attempts to explain its origin. Great damage was done by this perspective, greatly hindering the effective ministry of FBOs, for the first decades of HIV struggle. Consequently, much effort was made to educate and train FBOs towards compassion as exemplified by the WCC *Action Plan* (2002:6-7) for and by African churches, which made eradication of stigma its number one priority (see also the UNAIDS, *A Report of Theological Workshop Focusing on HIV and AIDS Related Stigma*). These efforts have borne good fruits, since several studies in Botswana indicate a significant move towards compassionate perspectives than stigmatization. For example, in his conclusion and recommendation chapter which appears in *Analysis of Clergy Views on Human Sexuality and HIV&AIDS Prevention: A Case Study of Mainline Churches* in Gaborone, Mussa Muneja points out that "churches have moved from being judgmental to being a welcoming abode for PLWHA, and other marginalized groups...However, the movement is not uniform, it varies from church to church and from clergy to clergy" (2006:151).

Nkomazana also holds that "Christian churches and church-related organizations are now committed to building up a compassionate community that responds to the needs of society in the midst of the AIDS epidemic. People living with HIV and AIDS are loved and accepted by God and are equal members of our community" (2007:67). Togarasei et. al (2008:9) found that "92% of participants were against stigmatization and discrimination of the infected and affected". An assessment carried by Dube during training of FBOs in Botswana on mainstreaming HIV and AIDS in the worship space also found that "there has been a shift from messages of stigmatization" but that "there is a scant attestation on messages of compassion" (Togarasei et al 2008:79).

The BNSF emphasizes the eradication of stigma and discrimination, mentioning it frequently in the activities of DMSACs (2003: 47, 48, 50, 51, 53, 55) but seldom were FBOs linked with the task of destigmatization, although one district sought "to "promote destigmatization at all levels— work, community, family and church." (55). Indeed the disassociation of FBOs with the role of reducing stigma and discrimination in the national response is perhaps best attested by *A Situational Analysis of Stigma Associated with HIV and AIDS: A Pilot Study* that hardly features or gives the views and activities of FBOs in destigmatization. Similarly, in the *Behaviour Change Interventions and Communications Strategy for the Health Sector (2006-2009),* HIV and AIDS stigma and discrimination is frequently featured (2005: 1, 27, 30 & 36) as an issue to be handled, yet FBOS are hardly associated with it. The national disassociation of FBOs with the role of destigmatization given the unfortunate response of FBOs towards HIV and AIDS are the beginning of the epidemic. Yet as the above studies highlight, FBOs have made a great move from stigma and discrimination towards compassion, solidarity, support and care for PLWHIV and the affected.

The MOH 2009 rapid assessment of FBOs response to HIV and AIDS confirms the findings of the above studies in the strongest terms. The study observes that:

> While the initial association of HIV and AIDS with sexual immorality led many FBOs to participate in HIV and stigma and discrimination, collected data and literature indicates that FBOs have made commendable strides towards compassion and support of PLWHA and the affected. Data indicates that there is unanimity among FBOs on the unacceptability of HIV stigma and discrimination and strong commitment to condemning any traces of all its forms. Indeed here, more than anywhere else, there was a general feeling of achievement and a happy commitment to further denounce traces of HIV stigma and discrimination (2009:59).

Documenting the methods used by FBOs to dispel stigma amongst their communities, the MOH 2009 rapid assessment found that:

> FBOs have used theological messages of compassion, acceptance, unity, loving and supporting one another to preach and teach against all forms of HIV and AIDS stigma and discrimination. FBOs also embarked on

concrete activities to discourage HIV and AIDS stigma and discrimination. These included such acts as visiting and caring for the PLWHA, eating with them, following up PLWHA that disappeared from fellowship and bringing them back, praying together and bringing PLWHA to a safety level, where they feel free to speak openly about their status. FBOs involved in physical healing (*Dingaka* and AICs) have used their healing services to reduce HIV stigma and discrimination by welcoming and attending PLWHA, a process that often involves washing and massaging clients (59).

Nonetheless, the study recommends that FBOs need to engage and involve more PLHWA and orphaned children in their programs. Indeed, this is particularly important to build the broken trust established by the FBOs' earlier response. Suspicion still lingers, not only among PLWHA, but also among the government workers, attested by the above mentioned strategies that do not associate FBOs with destigmatization. Botswana FBOs, on the other hand, are buoyant, confidently speaking in imperatives, "we don't allow" or "strongly against discrimination" (39).

Capacity Building

Capacity building is admittedly one of the weakest areas in the Botswana FBOs national response to HIV and AIDS given that FBOs are not profit making organizations and do not always have sufficient funds to sponsor training. Although HIV and AIDS now has 28 years of history, its multi-faceted complexity still calls for continued research and training and retraining. This is attested by various studies and reports. BOCAIP identifies challenges to be located in "skills in specialized areas." The Evangelical Fellowship of Botswana annual report points out that "the main challenge is to source funds to replicate the project to other districts. More efforts have to be added in fundraising and sustainability of the project" (Munamunungu 2008:27).

Turning to FBOs studies, Muneja's study, also sought to document "persisting limitations of the clergy on teaching about human sexuality and recommended training needs" (2006:152). The study made the following recommendations on training in:

1. counseling so as to mobilize their members to be HIV and AIDS competent in preventative approaches
2. biblical hermeneutics that will equip them to interpret scripture in empowering stance to all
3. gender sensitive issues to address gender imbalance (152-153).

In her report on training church leaders to mainstream HIV and AIDS
in worship, Dube lists the following capacity building needs, identified by
the FBO participants:

1. Further training on utilizing worship programs and space to
    respond to all aspects of HIV&AIDS is seriously needed, as
    strongly attested by all the three workshops.
2. Further encouragement and training of FBOs to utilize the HIV
    and AIDS calendar by planning for such days and months as
    December 1, Month of Youth Against HIV and AIDS, National
    Month of Prayer is needed.
3. Further training on a theology of compassion is needed. While
    the assessment indicates that there has been a shift from messages
    of stigmatization, there is scant attestation on messages of
    compassion. The WCC TEE module on compassion could come
    handy in this training.
4. Candle lighting service for breaking the stigma and healing
    (Togarasei et. al 2008:43), should be recommended for all
    churches/FBOs or even attached to a certain day in the church
    and HIV and AIDS calendar.
5. Translation of *AfricaPraying* into Setswana and other African
    languages is required.
6. Review of *AfricaPraying* to include the above suggestions would
    widen its targets and the utilization of more opportunities, which
    will be both national and international.
7. Further training on the content and use of *AfricaPraying,* which
    dedicates a full day to each part, that is, five days training
    workshops.
8. Production of the equivalent of *AfricaPraying* for other religions
    such as Islam and African Indigenous Religions would be very
    helpful" (2008: 78-79).

Following their assessment, T*ogarasei et. al.* (2008: 10-11) made the
following recommendations on training and empowerment of FBOs:

1. Provide FBOs with technical assistance in applying for funding,
    or developing proposals for HIV and AIDS related activities.
2. Provide opportunities for FBOs to hold regular regional and
    national meetings of umbrella faith-based organizations.
3. Improve or even develop IEC materials. These should be both in
    English and Setswana.

4. Empower HIV positive *Baruti* (pastors) and other FBOs leaders to go public with their status.
5. Organize HIV and AIDS training retreats for leaders or key personnel (training of trainers)
6. Help FBOs set up abstinence clubs for youth.
7. Empower women within FBOs, since they make things move. They are the majority FBOs.
8. Encourage FBOs to hold HIV testing days.
9. Conduct more research into AICs…whose beliefs and practices….deviate significantly from the other sub-categories of Christianity

The BNSF recognizes the need for building the capacity of FBOs, hence some DMSACs embraced the need to "educate traditional and religious leaders on HIV/AIDS prevention" (2003:49); "expand Home Based-Care services by establishing more hospices, counseling centers, clinics and building partnerships between government and non-government service providers" (53); "facilitate the development of programmes to economically empower the vulnerable groups in the district in conjunction with NGOs, the Private Sectors, headmen, churches and other stakeholders" (55); "support existing church programs to increase outreach to the infected and affected" (56) as well as calling for the "involvement of religious leaders in HIV/AIDS planning and activity implementation" (49). In general, the BNSF seems to emphasize the need to train traditional healers above all other FBOs.

Findings from the 2009 MOH rapid assessment of FBO's response to HIV and AIDS confirm the above studies.   According to the study:

The most common responses here (on capacity building) were, "Have not done much", "Need to do more". Generally umbrella organizations like BOCAIP are the ones that have done some capacity building work while most individual organizations have not done much and so noted this as a weakness. … For effective implementation of their HIV programmes, most FBOs called for training of pastors, volunteers, members, caregivers, PLWHA, vulnerable children and youth. Some AICs leaders also said their faith-healers, the poor and the unemployed need training in life skills and in HIV and AIDS issues. One respondent put is thus, "We need to be trained on how to deal with HIV/AIDS so that we know how to handle people with HIV without exposing ourselves to HIV." Mainstreaming of HIV and AIDS in theological training was also suggested (MOH 2009: 44 & 50).

Given that FBOs are non-profit making organizations; and that they do not always receive much support from donor agencies and governments, their limitations in capacity building are expected, but unfortunate, for they hinder FBOs from unleashing their full potential in the HIV and AIDS struggle. For example, among government officials, "There was a general consensus that the FBOs teachings on behavior change for abstinence and faithfulness are key to HIV prevention. Respondents argued that FBOs are the best sector to promote behavior change… . All they need are resources and training on how best to influence behavior change through the values of their specific faiths" (53).

Closing Remarks

FBOs are amongst the oldest institutions that we have in Botswana. Their service to the Divine often provides the strongest foundation for supporting life and justice. Although fallible, as attested by their unfortunate history of stigmatizing, FBOs still provide the best front for HIV and AIDS response in the areas of prevention, care, support, treatment, de-stigmatizing, advocacy, networking and behavior change. Yet given that FBOs are not profit making, they are not always the best resourced in terms of finances, capacity building and monitoring. However, given that they are passionate about protecting life and treating all life as sacred, it is a social capital that takes them far. This means that many professionals in their midst are willing to volunteer their skills; many rich people are willing to give lots of money and other resources to FBOs; many members are willing to volunteer their times to care for orphans and visit the sick while religious leaders enjoy the trust of the community, which makes their messages better received. FBOs, in their fallibility, represent the hope for life that the Creator has given to all of us. In the national response to HIV and AIDS, FBOs represent a friend who will always walk with us. For example, in the MOH 2009 rapid assessment of Botswana FBOs, one aspect that undeniably shines through is the FBOs' passion for staying the course in the HIV and AIDS struggle. FBOs thus remain a sign of hope pointing us to the God with us even in the troubling times. FBOs' strength lies in their broad commitment to the sacredness of life and people as a whole. One cannot over-emphasize that:

> FBOs operate in parallel to governments providing virtually all the same major services as the government but filling in the gaps where government fails to provide. Their outreach activities are to be found contributing to virtually every institution, including medical, education, social welfare and justice and peace. Support for orphans and vulnerable children extends

from community based initiatives to institutional care. They also offer care in correctional facilities, poverty alleviation schemes, agricultural projects, feeding programs, homeless shelters and support for the street children and are widely involved in development work. When government services fail, FBOs are increasingly being asked to back up and support previously functioning systems (Parry 2003: 14).

More support from other stakeholders and networking in the HIV and AIDS struggle, such as donor communities and government is needed to assist FBOs perform their best in the national HIV and AIDS response. More investment into FBOs' capacity to engage in the HIV and AIDS struggle is no doubt a mustard seed that is sown in a fertile soil for the greater well being of the whole society.

Bibliography

Amadiume, I. *Male Daughters, Female Husbands.* London: Zed Books, 1987.
—. *Re-inventing Africa: Matriarchy, Religion and Culture.* London: ZED Books, 1997.
Ampomah, K. "Collaborative Approaches Within Church Networks and UNAIDS," In *Come Let us Rebuild: Faith Based HIV/AIDS Summit 1-5TH Dec, 2003.* Gaborone, Botswana Christian Council, 2005, 39-41.
ARHAP. *Working at the Intersection of Religion and Public Health: A Bounded Field of Unknowing.* Cape Town: ARPHAP – UCT, 2005.
BCC, *Adolescents Sexual Health.* Gaborone: BCC, 2003.
BOCAIP, 'Botswana Christian AIDS Intervention Program: A Christian Response to HIV/AIDS in Botswana,' (unpublished power point presentation).
Botswana Population and Housing Census, Gaborone: Central Statistics Office, 2001.
Chitando, E. *Living and Acting with Hope Vol. 1 and 2,* Geneva: WCC Publications, 2007.
—. *Living with Hope: African Churches and HIV/AIDS Volume 1.* Geneva: WCC, 2007.
CMRS, *Forward in Hope: A Plan of Action for the Next Twelve Months: A Response to HIV/AIDS By the Joint Conference of Major Religious Superiors in Zimbabwe.* Harare: Health Desk, 2005.
Cochrane , J. and B. Schimd (Eds.). *ARHAP Tools: Workshop Report.* Cape Town: UCT, 2004.
Dube, M. W. (ed.), *HIV/AIDS and the Curriculum: Methods of Integrating HIV/AIDS in Theological Programs.* Geneva: WCC, 2003.

—. *The HIV and AIDS Bible: Selected Essays.* Scranton: Scranton University Press, 2008.

—. "Training Faith Leaders in Mainstreaming HIV&AIDS into the Worship Programs and Spaces," in L. Togarasei et. al. *An Assessment of the Capacity of Faith-Based Organizations for HIV Prevention in Botswana.* Gaborone: Associated Press, 2008, 77-79.

—. *AfricaPraying: A Handbook on HIV/AIDS Sensitive Sermon and Liturgy.* Geneva: WCC, 2003.

—. *Theology in the HIV and AIDS Context: A Series of Ten Distant Learning Modules* (in CD form). Geneva: WCC, 2008.

—. "Rebuilding Botswana: The Gospel and the Challenge and HIV&AIDS," In *Come Let us Rebuild: Faith Based HIV/AIDS Summit 1-5TH Dec, 2003.* Gaborone, Botswana Christian Council, 2005, 49-63.

—. (Ed). *Other Ways of Reading: African Women and the Bible,* Atlanta: SBL, 2001.

Gaie, J. B. R. and Mmolai, S. K. (eds.). *The Concept of Botho and HIV/AIDS in Botswana.* Eldoret: ZAPF Chancery, 2007.

Haron M. et. al "Ditumelo Secondary Literature Review: HIV Prevention and Faith-Based Organisation in Botswana." In *BOLESWA Journal of Theology, Religion and Philosophy,* Volume 2:1, 2008, 1-64.

Landmann, C. "Spiritual Care-Giving to Women affected by HIV/Aids." In Phiri I. A., Haddad, B. and Masenya, M. (eds.). *African Women, HIV/Aids and Faith Communities.* Pietermaritzburg: Cluster Press, 2003, 189-208.

Ministry of Health,.*Behaviour Change Interventions and Communication Strategy for Health Sector (2006-2009).* Gaborone: Ministry of Health, 2006.

—. *Botswana ANC Second Generation HIV/AIDS Sentinel Surveillance Technical Report.* Gaborone: Ministry of Health, undated.

—. *Action Plan for People with Disability and HIV/AIDS in Botswana* (2005-2007). Gaborone: Ministry of Health, 2005.

—. *Botswana Safe Male Circumcision: Add-on Strategy for HIV Prevention.* Gaborone: Ministry of Health, 2008.

—. *Rapid Assessment for FBOs HIV&AIDS Strategy Development.* Gaborone: MOH, (unpublished report), 2009 .

Ministry of Local Government, *National Situational Analysis on Orphans and Vulnerable Children in Botswana.* Gaborone, Ministry of Local Government, 2008.

—. *National Situational Analysis on Orphans and Vulnerable Children in Botswana.* Gaborone, Ministry of Local Government, 2008.

Modiega, D. "Keynote Address," In *Come Let us Rebuild: Faith Based HIV/AIDS Summit 1-5TH Dec, 2003.* Gaborone, Botswana Christian Council, 22-28.

MTP II 1997-2002. *Botswana HIV and AIDS: 2nd Medium Term Plan.* Gaborone: Ministry of Health, 1997.

Munamunungu, M. (undated). *Evangelical Fellowship of Botswana HIV/AIDS Initiative—Reaching Out to the Communities 2005-2008.* (Unpublished report).

Muneja, M. *An Analysis of Church Clergy Views on Human Sexuality and HIV&AIDS: A Case Study of Churches in Gaborone.* unpublished MA thesis, Gaborone: University of Botswana, 2006.

NACA. *Botswana National Strategic Framework for HIV&AIDS 2003-2009.* Gaborone: Pyramid Publishing, 2003.

—. *Botswana AIDS Impact Survey III, Preliminary Results,* Gaborone: Central Statistics Office, 2009.

—. *National Strategy for Behaviour Change Interventions and Communications for HIV and AIDS.* Gaborone: NACA, 2006.

—. *Progress Report on the National Response to the UNGASS Declaration of Commitment on HIV/AIDS.* Gaborone: NACA, 2008.

—. *National Operational Plan for Scaling Up HIV and AIDS in Botswana.* Gaborone: NACA, 2008.

Nkomazana   F. "Christian Ethics and HIV/AIDS in Botswana," In Amanze, J. (ed.).   *Christian Ethics and HIV/AIDS in Africa.* Gaborone: Bay Publishing, 2007, 48-69.

Parry, S. *Responses of the Faith-Based Organizations to HIV/Aids in Sub-Saharan Africa.* Geneva: WCC, 2003.

The Botswana Guardian, 25 May 2007.

Togarasei, L. et. al. *An Assessment of the Capacity of Faith-Based Organizations for HIV Prevention in Botswana.* Gaborone: Associated Printers, 2008.

Togarasei, L. *Rapid Assessment Report for FBOs Strategy.* Ministry of Health, Botswana, 2009.

Vision 2016, *Long Term Vision for Botswana—Towards Prosperity for All.* Gaborone: Government Printers, 1997.

Yang, D. J. "Prevention: Protecting Life," In *Come Let us Rebuild: Faith Based HIV/AIDS Summit 1-5TH Dec, 2003.* Gaborone: Botswana Christian Council, 2005, 15.

WCC, *Plan of Action: The Ecumenical Response to HIV&AIDS.* Geneva: WCC, 2001.

www.wikpedia.org/wiki/faith-based

CHAPTER THREE

THE POLITICS OF FAITH-BASED HIV PREVENTION POLICIES AND PROGRAMS IN BOTSWANA

KIPTON E. JENSEN

"The AIDS industry is a prisoner of political circumstance, and as a result, may be trapped in a cycle of ineffectiveness" (de Waal 2003: 255).

Introduction

Although the global public health community has made significant advances in understanding the biology of the human immunodeficiency virus (HIV), as well as developing reliable diagnostic tests and effective drugs for prolonging the life of the infected, the rate of transmission and – in the case of Botswana – the prevalence rate remains alarmingly high. Part of the explanation for this alleged ineffectiveness, itself a point of contention, may have less to do with the attitudes or behaviours of Batswana than with the politics of public health prevention policies adopted by Botswana (Heald 2002, de Cock 2002, de Waal 2003, Allen and Heald 2004; Green, Halperin, Nantulya and Hogle 2006). And while Botswana is often hailed as an exception to the rule in sub-Saharan Africa, what de Waal (2003:255) claims for Africa – namely, that "the AIDS industry is a prisoner of political circumstance" – is perhaps doubly true when applied to Botswana.

Following a concise history of Botswana's response to HIV and AIDS, this essay explores the political circumstances that have haunted if not imprisoned HIV prevention programs in general and faith-based initiatives in particular. Unfortunately, there remain numerous hindrances to religious collaboration: e.g., the "identity politics" of HIV Prevention programs and policies in Botswana, including "international versus Indigenous systems of knowledge and discourse of power," the politics of religious identity, both theoretically and practically, the "faith politics" of HIV prevention programs (Government Organizations and Non Governmental Organizations), as well as theoretical and practical inducements against "inter-sectoral" and "intra-sectoral" collaboration.

Country Profile and Response Timeline

Botswana has one of the highest infection rates worldwide: it is estimated that 350,000 Batswana (20% of the total population of 1.765 million) have been infected (CDC, 2006). The incidence is higher in selected population groups, such as, pregnant women (37.4%), 15-19 year olds (30%) and those between the ages of 20 and 24 years (50%). The World Health Organization estimates life expectance at 40 years, down from 61 years before the pandemic; a further decrease to 33 years is expected by the year 2010. The nation has approximately 67,000 AIDS orphans (CDC, 2006). Across the spectrum of age groups, suggests the latest estimates (BIAS II), approximately 17% of the population is HIV+. In the worst hit health districts, districts to the north and west, prevalence exceeds 40% for both men and women between 15 and 49. Infection is distributed unequally between men and women, of course, with women carrying more than their share of the burden, and the poor in towns are hit hardest. Young women are at higher risk of HIV infection than their male counterparts: the prevalence among women aged 15-19 years was 9.8 percent versus 3.1 percent of men of the same age (CDC 2006).

Because of the relatively early detection of HIV within the population, a quick national response (National Emergency Plan 1987) and committed leaders (for example former President, Festus Mogae), early VCT and free ART (2001) programs, as well as dedicated international donors and a strong medical infrastructure, and all of this within a country that is both democratic and economically stable, "one might have supposed that if western AIDS policies were capable of working anywhere in Africa they should have worked here" (Heald 2005: 5). And while there are some who claim that western-based prevention strategies have been, "in the main, signally ineffective" (Heald 2005: 2) in Africa, Botswana has achieved success – arguably significant success – in its partnership with international health agencies: 84% of new antenatal care clients were tested as part of the national PMTCT program, mother to child transmission has dropped from an estimated 16% to less than 4%, almost 100% awareness of HIV, relatively high levels of reported condom use with non-cohabiting partners (76%), and Botswana was one of the first countries in Africa to introduce routine HIV-testing policies.   Yet, prevalence rates remain high. How is one to explain the seeming success of prevention programs in Uganda, for example, to draw on a comparison often discussed in recent literature strategy (Epstein 2004, 2005; Halperin, et al 2004; Stoneburner and Low-Beer 2004; Hearst and Chen 2004; Green 2003, 2006; Shelton, 2005; Wilson 2004; Cohen 2004), a regional neighbor who lacked the structural advantages afforded our beloved Botswana? And how is one to explain the *alleged or prima facie* failure of prevention programs in Botswana despite its structural largesse (relative to other countries in the region)?

The "Identity Politics" of HIV Prevention Programs in Botswana: International versus Indigenous Methods and Programs.

It would oversimplify the present public health campaign to treat the standard ABC prevention message, which is not so much a message as a collection of three very important facts about barriers to HIV transmission, as constituting the mainstay of prevention efforts in Botswana. But it does seem that the Government reached out to international experts, in good faith, from the beginning: adopting the ABC educational message, and perhaps even stressing the C of the message, Botswana's approach was also informed by lessons learned from abroad about the importance of testing and stigmatization and the dangers of violating of human rights. This approach seemed to be imminently reasonable. And yet, as Heald captures so well in the following observations, first in 2004 and later in 2005,

> [t]he Government's following of an exclusively western model fuelled suspicion, which the exclusion of diviners, healers, and churchmen from the campaigns did nothing to ameliorate. Two parallel discourses existed, one official and one non-official, and this latter in the absence of any recognition had the potential to take on decidedly politial overtones (Heald 2004: 1145; also see Ingstad 2001).

> The HIV prevention campaign in Botswana challenged the old arbiters of truth, who found their values and assumptions over-ridden or ignored. In contrast to surrounding countries, traditional doctors, churchmen and local communities were not incorporated into the educational effort. It was exclusively in the hands of official channels and thus to a large extent seen as 'external' or white – i.e., *sekgoa* as opposed to *setswana* (Heald 2005: 6).

In reference to the UNAIDS/WHO HIV epidemiological sheets, Chilisa also detects

> . . . a naming game where those with the highest HIV/AIDS prevalence rates in the world, like Botswana, increasingly come under pressure to embrace Western-prescribed norms, buy the circulating knowledge and technology on HIV/AIDS, and sacrifice the vulnerable sick to research experiments and drug trials. The research on HIV/AIDS simply works within the colonially established framework of homogeneity in the search for answers and solutions to the HIV/AIDS pandemic. This leaves out the voices of the researched 'other,' namely the former colonized languages and cultures (2005: 667).

This is a serious challenge to international collaboration, a principled objection, sometimes discussed under the banner of "nothing for Africa, without Africa." To suggest that public health programs and policies are not unrelated to post-colonial identity politics, which constitutes a principled insistence on respecting the indigenous voices, is instructive. One need not cite Foucault's formula that power resides in the authority to control the terms of what counts as "legitimate discourse," or good science, nor even Airhihenbuwa's *Health and Culture: Beyond the Western Paradigm*, to see the inter-personal "othering" inherent in addressing a public health crisis. But what are the costs, opportunity costs included, of this admittedly legitimate and principled objection to if not an obstacle to a more effective collaborative strategy? Is there a way past this hindrance to improved collaboration?

In her "What has Worked in Uganda and Failed in Botswana," written with Tim Allen, Heald (2004) argues that Uganda emphasized A and B while Botswana emphasized condoms and neglected abstinence and fidelity. In 2002, already, Heald declared that the failure of AIDS intervention strategies aimed at prevention in Botswana and other African countries, by which she means Western approaches, is no longer in doubt. One of the reasons, she argues, is "a lack of cultural sensitivity." Green and Halerpin, et al (2006), as well as Epstein (2004, 2005a), seem to agree with Heald that Western intervention strategies have failed; the only real dispute is why it didn't work and who is to blame. What remains, however, after the finger-pointing game is concluded, is to suggest a more effective alternative. Amidst the blame game, people are still dying for a more culturally sensitive or otherwise more effective approach. She also argues that the ABC message, which is "the language of western science and policy," is neither universally relevant nor morally neutral. It is also founded, she says, on a misguided model of rational choice – namely,

. . . that given the facts and presented with alternatives, people will act with
self-preservation in mind. This theory, as we have all come to know, is
deeply flawed: Human choices are constrained and depend on who and
where one is, especially in such an emotive and important an area as
human sexuality. People cannot be assumed to be autonomous agents
operating in a vacuum (Allen and Heald 2004: 2-3).

If Western models of behavioral change are based on a distinctively
Western conception of the self, and if Batswana operate according to a
unique if not distinctively non-Western notion of the self, then the
adaption of Western models of behavior change to Botswana are doomed
to ineffectiveness (see Gaie and Jensen, 2008). In short, writes Heald,
"[t]he message is read not as about a neutral scientific 'fact' but as a
rejection of morality and of culture" (3). The Government AIDS message
then is seen as politically loaded: it is "not promulgating a universal truth
but a sectional Western (White) one" (Heald 2004:3). In contemporary
constructivist thought, writes Petraglia (2009: 177), "cognition is not an
abstract, purely symbolic manipulation of data but a process embedded in
our everyday interactions with the world, interactions that are always
mediated by language or symbols."

Petraglia, who worked with the *Makgabaneng* radio program in
Botswana, goes on to suggest that "[l]anguage is the means by which we
'share' and 'distribute' cognition . . . This perspective on learning takes
the focus off the thinker in isolation and asks what we look to everyday
activity as a source of information; we think in conjunction with our
perceptions of the world around us" (2009:177). Critics of Western models
of HIV prevention in Botswana ask us to consider the consequences of
using imported frameworks of knowledge in the struggle against HIV and
AIDS. From the postcolonial framework, argues Chilisa (2005: 680), HIV
prevention in Botswana "has been highly compromised by employing
language and categories of thinking that are alien to the infected and
affected communities." This alienation is not unavoidable. As a case in
point, Ingstad claims that the categorization of HIV, either as a Tswana
ailment or a modern disease, "may have important consequences for
prevention. Advocating condoms as a way to prevent *meila* probably
carries more incentive than advocating them to prevent pregnancy or other
sexual transmitted diseases" (2002:7). There is – once one gets beyond
the territorialism – a striking similarity between ideas of disease
transmission in the Tswana medical system and notions of AIDS
transmission in biomedicine. "In both conceptual systems," writes Ingstad,
"sexual intercourse, blood, and transmission from mothers to their babies

play a role. Also in both systems disease or AIDS is strongly associated with sexual rules of society" (Ingstad 1990: 83).

The Politics of Religious Identity in Botswana: *O wa tumelo efe?*

Religious identity is one hindrance to effective collaboration in HIV response in Botswana. From the outset, religious identity in Botswana has been politically charged. Indeed, religious freedom is a relatively new phenomenon, something constitutionally guaranteed only at the time of independence (1966). Because LMS missionaries were political assets, especially in their role in assuring protectorate status for Botswana and from expansionists from both South Africa and Rhodesia between 1904 and 1924, these missionaries were often granted exclusive permission to evangelize on the condition that they offer medical care and education. This is particularly true of the Khama realm. Other religious traditions, or even different denominations within Protestantism, were denied access to most territories. One religion, some argued, is enough; more than one will lead to schisms. Though many chiefs were deferential to LMS missionaries, they were also closely monitored: at times, the power struggle for authority was bitter, at other times it was merely a subtext to privilege. Though Kgosi Khama viewed himself as head of the Church, many missionaries challenged the indigenous authority and appealed to chiefs to subvert other loci of authority – e.g., traditional healers and initiation rites. The LMS did not approve of ordination for Batswana, something that eventually led to the establishment – often underground – of the first AICs.

Translating the Bible into Setswana demonstrates the political struggle of missionaries to root out traditional cultural practices and beliefs that they considered contrary to the Christian faith – e.g., 'ancestors' was translated as 'evil spirits.' Traditional healers were accused of practicing witchcraft [*boloi*], and missionaries aggressively lobbied to have non-deferential *Dingaka* imprisoned or otherwise banned. In many cases, religious conflict was politically motivated and had political consequences (see Dube 1999, Ntloedibe-Kuswani 2003). Male circumcision was standard practice, as part of the male initiation rites, prior to the arrival of the missionaries. As it turns out, male circumcision has been proven to reduce the risk of HIV transmission in men by approximately 60 per cent (UNAIDS Epidemic Update 2006, "Male circumcision: Africa's unprecedented opportunity").

The religious identity question was first included in the national census in 1946, at a time when Botswana was still known as Bechuanaland. At that point, there were but two possible responses: Animist or Christian. From the outset, it seems safe to say, religious identity in Botswana "has been more political than evangelical." The question was dropped from subsequent surveys circulated in 1956, 1964, 1971, 1981 and 1991 (Damschke & Goyer: 1986). The Central Statistics Office reintroduced the religious identity question as part of the 2001 Botswana Population and Housing Census. According to the 2001 Botswana census, which surveyed 1,189,688 citizens, the dominant religious tradition in Botswana was Christianity (852,160 or 72%), followed by *Badimo* (71,329 or 6%), Muslim (5,036), Hindu (3,017), and numerous minority faith communities (e.g., Buddhism, Sikhism, Bahai, and Judaism); 244,832 (21%) citizens considered themselves non-religious. The question posed in the census was "What is your religion?" The categories offered were: (1) Christian, (2) Muslim, (3) Bahai, (4) Hindu, (5) Badimo, (6) Other, and (7) No religion. It is often noted that "*badimo*" inadequately represents 'African traditional religions,' since the veneration of the ancestors is but one specific article of faith – e.g., the virgin birth of Christ or the authority of the Pope – rather than a complex religious tradition.

Prior to the release of the 2001 census data, however, most scholars estimated that a significantly higher proportion of Batswana belonged to traditional African religious traditions (hereafter ATR). In 1994, Amanze suggested that 80% of religious Batswana belonged to traditional African religions and only 20% were Christian. Nkomazana estimated in 2001 that approximately 65% were 'traditional indigenous religion' and 35% were Christian (2001: 341). In 2002, Melton claimed that approximately 40% of Batswana were 'ethno-religious' – defined as "adherents of local, tribal or shamanistic practices" – and 60% were Christian. The 2003 BAIS II study reported that 82 % of Batswana are Christian, 4% belong to 'badimo' religious traditions, 12 % claimed to have 'no religion,' and that all other religious categories – Islam, Hinduism, and other – constituted less than 2 % of the population. Compared to the estimates provided by Amanze (1994), Nkomazana (1998, 2001a) and Melton (2002), the BAIS II information seems to confirm the relative accuracy of the 2001 Census data. In a recent albeit relatively small survey, Population Studies International (PSI: 2006a) reported that 72% of their respondents identified themselves as Christian (9% AIC, and 63% 'other Christian'), 4% 'traditionalist' and 23% as claiming 'no religion' (PSI: 2006).

The discrepancies in estimates, as well as surveillance results, are puzzling. In his "Botswana's Population Census 2001: An Analysis and

Interpretation of its different Religious Traditions", Haron (2004: 334) argues that the

> Batswana [religious] identity seems to be fluid when it comes to Christianity and African traditional religions; there exists a marriage of convenience to the extent that individuals belong to both the church and the ATR at the same time, and because of this situaticn, the figures fluctuate dramatically between the two categories.

And indeed, these two categories are themselves inadequately if not inconsistently defined. But apart from questions cf academic or demographic categorization, the issue of religious identity is – often, though not always – a real point of contention (see Haron & Jensen: 2007). During the colonial period, e.g., and for shrewd political reasons, writes Ngwenya (2001) "chiefs actively promoted Christianity and banned traditional African religions and African-initiated churches . . . which were perceived as posing a threat to central authority and social rank" (also Landau 1997; Comaroff & Comaroff 1997; Elphick 1998; Ntloedibe-Kuswani 2003). Batswana are often syncretistic in their religious orientation, which means that they interweave or stack religious traditions.

The most radical proposed re-categorization of religious identity, one rooted in the "surprising" estimate that 12% of Batswana (BAIS II) claimed that they do not have a religion, is that "in Africa one is born religious; by being born African and continue to live as an African, one remains an African religionist" (Ntloedibe-Kuswani 2003). On this model of categorization, the religious identity question loses its value: since the BAIS II survey is designed exclusively for citizens of Botswana, almost all of whom were "born in Africa and continue to live as an African," all or almost all respondents should – following the *de facto* Ntloedibe-Kuswani proposal – be viewed as "African religionists." Despite their espoused religious affiliations, suggests Ntloedibe-Kuswani, Batswana "remain Africans [and thus belong primarily to ATR] though they have also identified with foreign religions." This argument makes a good though perhaps exaggerated point. As a demographic variable, religious identity may well be useful as a guide to developing more effective national policies and programs. And yet, Ntloedibe-Kuswani is not alone in asserting that the "failure to recognize the uniqueness of African religions, or the Batswana religion, has resulted in African and the Batswana having lost their identity (*Boleng*) as well as their humanness (*Botho*)" (see Setiloane, 1978; Chilisa, 2005). Indeed, Ntloedibe-Kuswani suggests that "[t]he colonising nature of some non-indigenous religious traditions has incapacitated or emasculated (*go kgaetsa*) many Batswana not to fully recognise their own as authentic and fulfilled" (2003: 3). For many Batswana, however, Christianity constitutes a new identity, one that implies a conscious if not explicit rejection of the past (see Togarasei 2006). Is it true that indigenous religious traditions have been "marginalized or ridiculed out of existence through colonial intervention?" At what point, culturally or historically, might Christianity also qualify as an indigenous religious phenomenon? African Independent Churches, sometimes called African Indigenous Churches, would certainly disagree with those who argue that the only way to be genuinely African is to reject all so-called 'foreign religions.' Indeed, it could even be argued that Christianity – at least in its Augustinian formulation – is indigenous to Africa.

For the purposes of the present chapter, however, the simple point is that religious identity is itself politically charged. It is unclear whether questions of religious identity present a possible hindrance to inter-religious, even ecumenical, collaboration with respect to HIV prevention programs and policies as well as inter-sectoral collaboration. There are, suggest Gerrie Ter Haar and Stephen Ellis (2006: 353), "eminently practical reasons for including religion with the broad concept of development" – under the auspices of which we might include HIV prevention and care – because "religion, whatever form it takes, constitutes a social and political reality."

The "Faith Politics" of HIV Prevention Programs: Inter-Sectoral and Intra-Sectoral (Non-) Collaboration.

As a working assumption, enhanced collaboration amongst religious communities as well as collaboration between religious communities and the Government of Botswana Ministry of Health is important to achieving the shared task of turning the tide on HIV infection in Botswana. But there are looming obstacles to enhancing collaboration on both of these fronts: the initial public health discourse was at least initially incongruent with the indigenous discourse concerning the HIV ailment, both culturally and religiously, some traditionalists are non-cooperative as a matter of cultural principle, and faith communities can occasionally become rather competitive when it comes to winning congregants or adherents. And indeed, intra-sectoral non-cooperation is sometimes the result of long-standing theological if not also political disagreements between religious communities.

In questions of human rights and social justice, communities of faith have often been found at the frontlines. But in the present HIV and AIDS crisis, at least in southern Africa, the hardest hit region of the epidemic, the civil sector in general and faith-oriented communities in particular have been – it is sometimes suggested – curiously slow to respond. And stigmatization within faith communities, even within leadership, remained an ongoing concern for a long time. Though many communities of faith claim to be 'ready to join arms in the fight against HIV and AIDS in Africa' (see Togarasei et al: 2008), examples of effective ecumenical collaboration are often inconspicuous. Why is that? Is faith important or even decisive to promoting healthy behaviours? Are ecumenical collaborations important or even decisive to combating HIV?

Obstacles to "inter-sectoral collaboration"

The initial disagreement between these two sectors, public health and the faith sector, arose as the response of "churchmen" to the inclusion of barrier methods, especially "condomization," as part of the HIV prevention message. Objecting as Christians as well as traditional Batswana, church leaders were indignant with public health officials who spoke with their children about protective sex in schools, incensed when radio messages and billboards were introduced as part of the governmental HIV prevention campaign, and enflamed when those officials approved public health programs on how to correctly and safely unwrap and apply a condom. Following Ingstad (2001), Heald (2005) claims:

> The promotion of barrier methods to prevent infection set up the cry of immorality, of encouraging promiscuity. As such, it met with the resistance of churches, parents and population. This disbelief of the facts and the opposition in terms of morality fed in and fuelled an alternative discourse of AIDS, which grew out of Tswana beliefs and understanding. . . . In effect, one had two parallel discourses operating: one was government endorsed and public, making the second appear as the unofficial and sub rosa, though for many it was these truths that appeared self-evident (Heald 2005: 5-6).

These parallel discourses constitute a residual obstacle to the development of a collaborative inter-sectoral prevention strategy. It is worth noting, though, that these allegedly parallel discourses are not irreconcilable. Kealotswe (2001: 221) suggests that members of AICs tended to classify AIDS as a form of *boswagadi*, "which is believed to attack a man who has had sexual intercourse with a widow who had not been properly purified after the death of her husband" (also Ingstad 1990 and Heald 2004, 2005). Whereas Kealotswe argues that "the absence of a traditional Batswana concept of disease by means of which to interpret HIV/AIDS is one of the causes of its rapid spread, because many people cannot be convinced of the existence of a mysterious disease that has no equivalent in their world view" (2001: 221), Ingstad observes "a striking similarity between ideas of disease transmission and *meila* in the Tswana medical system and notions of AIDS transmission in biomedicine" (1990: 33).

At the functional level of behavior change, both discourses acknowledge that HIV is contracted through unsafe forms of sexual intercourse, at least primarily, and that one must become properly purified of the blood ailment before one can responsibly have sex with another person. In both discourses, abstinence – until one knows all the relevant facts and, if appropriate, receives the prescribed treatment of a healer – is advised; both discourses advise, to greater or lesser degrees, sexual fidelity within monogamous relationships. If abstinence before marriage and fidelity within marriage, ideally between concordant couples, were adhered to faithfully, then the promotion of barrier methods to prevent infection would be unnecessary. Traditionalists and indigenous church leaders sometimes suggested that the promotion of condoms was unnecessary, even counter-productive, since the message that one could protect oneself with a condom is motivationally inconsistent with the advice to abstain (or, for married couples, to remain faithful to one another). And indeed, Uganda adopted a relatively successful HIV prevention strategy of abstinence and fidelity only, i.e., without publicly endorsing condom use. Green et al (2006: 342) suggest that while it

> . . . makes good epidemiological sense to address all three ABC behaviors rather than to promote only one or two components of 'ABC,' a great deal of resources have gone into primarily biomedical-based interventions (i.e., VCT, STI treatment, condoms) in South Africa, Botswana and other southern African countries, yet without apparent impact on national HIV infection rates (see also Allen and Heald, 2004; Epstein, 2004; Green 2003; Hearst and Chen, 2004; Wilson, 2004).

The good news is that Botswana's public health strategy has had an apparent, albeit modest, impact on national HIV infection and prevalence rates. The 2009 AIDS Epidemic Update reported that new HIV infections have been slashed by 17 per cent globally (UNAIDS, 2009); the adult HIV prevalence rate shows signs of declining in urban areas (UNAIDS, 2009). Also, "the percentage of 20–24-year-old antenatal clinic attendees who were HIV-infected in Botswana fell from 38.7% in 2001 to 27.9% in 2007 (Botswana Ministry of Health, 2008). But the question looms whether "the success [of Uganda] can be replicated elsewhere in Africa (not to mention in very different, more concentrated epidemics such as those in Asia or Latin America)" (ibid.).

To be sure, there are substantial points of inter-sectoral agreement between communities of faith and the public health community with respect to HIV prevention. Above all else, both sectors are committed – usually with great passion – to a shared and undeniably good goal: to reduce the risk and impact of HIV and AIDS. Both sectors are stressing abstinence and fidelity, and many communities of faith are not shy about discussing the importance of responsible condom use (Togarasei et al: 2008). Most communities of faith, like the HIV and AIDS health community, promote testing and adherence to ART. Communities of faith in Botswana are trying to address the unjust social conditions that contribute to the epidemic (Togarasei et al: 2008). Both sectors are working against, in word if not in deed, stigmatization. Both sectors are speaking out against alcohol and drug abuse. Beyond stressing the need for prevention messages, the public health community and faith-based organizations are trying to alleviate suffering associated with HIV and AIDS by caring for orphans and vulnerable children as well as providing hospice care and counseling. Both agree that prevention, especially behavior change and a more just system, is the best defense against the ills associated with HIV and AIDS. In both discourses, the ailment of HIV is associated with inappropriate or unsafe sexual intercourse, or exchange of blood, they both advise abstinence until sanctioned by a medical practitioner, fidelity within marriage, and it is recognized as a disease quite unlike those traditionally encountered. There is also a shared notion, between traditional healers and bio-medical practitioners, that treatment is often a matter of controlling the symptoms rather than curing the ailment or disease. But there is a good deal of disagreement between sectors on the value and effects of condom use in preventing HIV. There is, in short, common ground to be found between traditional medical practitioners, as well as spiritual healers and church communities, and government-sponsored public health officials. But there remain substantial – though not insurmountable – obstacles to both inter-sectoral and intra-sectoral collaboration when it comes to serving those who are suffering. Ultimately, these obstacles – whether they constitute minor or major differences, whether animated by narcissism or loyalty – must be transformed into a call to service.

Intra-sectoral Collaboration as a pre-requisite
to Inter-sectoral Collaboration

It would oversimplify the matter to assume that the various faith communities that comprise the faith-sector in Southern Africa, from traditional African religions and mainline Christianity to Islam and Independent African Churches, share a common faith or universal creed or shared set of rituals or symbolic language or attitude or knowledge system or behavior or strategies for changing behavior and social accountability or even an unbiased appreciation of what other faith communities believe and say about HIV and AIDS (Togarasei et al: 2008). Perhaps the sole common denominator is that the HIV epidemic puts our respective faiths, each in its own way, to the test. And while national public health policies, e.g., the *Botswana National Strategic Framework*, often call for multi-sectoral approaches, in which various sectors join arms, it will be difficult to achieve an effective inter-sectoral collaboration between, e.g., the public health sector and the faith sector, if there is a failure to effectively cooperate across denominational – not to mention ecumenical – lines within the faith sector itself.

Responses to HIV, as well as HIV prevention messages and programs, differ considerably across denominations and faith traditions (see Togarasei et al: 2008); and yet they tend to agree that the best advice is that people should abstain from sex until marriage and remain faithful within marriage. It is fairly common to characterize if not caricature churches in Botswana, as elsewhere, not only in sub-Saharan Africa, as 'anti-condom.' And while it is true that many faith communities oppose the use of condoms, usually because it detracts from the primary message of abstinence until marriage and fidelity within marriage, it is less true of African Independent Churches than it is of – for example – Pentecostal churches. Although many faith communities consider themselves to be well-aligned to the ABC slogan of HIV prevention, the emphasis has been on abstinence and faithfulness at the expense of condomising. Until recently, church leaders tended to promote condom use for those who cannot abstain nor be faithful to their HIV negative married partners. Along these lines, it is not uncommon for faith leaders to suggest that: *Sekausu se diritswe batho ba ba sa kgoneng go itshoka, fa o sa kgone o ka se dirisa* (i.e., that condoms were made for those who cannot restrain themselves from sexual intercourse). This hierarchicalization of the A-B-C message within most faith communities, where risk avoidance is promoted above risk reduction, is important. Togarasei et al (2008) note that from district workshop discussions it was clear that faith leaders want to avoid sending a mixed message – i.e., that their congregants should abstain on the one hand but carry a condom in their wallet or purse on the other. The promotion of barrier methods to reduce the risk of infection by the Ministry of Health in Botswana, following an epidemiological model based on the experience of AIDS in the United States, writes Heald (2005: 5), "set up the cry of immorality, of encouraging promiscuity. As such, it met with the resistance of churches, parents and population." And while Heald captures nicely the political dimension of the initial HIV prevention campaign in Botswana, from their study, Togarasei et al (2008) suggest that the characterization of churches as 'anti-condom' has changed over time and that the view of condoms varies considerably between denominations. The study shows that across faith communities, 40% of the survey respondents claimed that the leadership had promoted condom use among the unmarried members of the faith community within sermons or formal teachings. When the responses were disaggregated along denominational lines, the survey found that promoting condom use among unmarried couples within congregations varies significantly: Whereas only 12% of the respondents from Pentecostal churches said that they promoted condom use among unmarried couples from the pulpit, and approximately 36% from mainline churches, approximately 73% of the respondents from AICs said that they promoted condom use among unmarried couples from the pulpit within the past six months. Asked differently, the survey asked respondents whether their commitment to promoting condom use among unmarried couples was "very strong" or "strong" or "weak." The contrast between AICs and Pentecostal churches was significant: whereas 67% of AICs described their commitment level as very strong or strong, only 18% of Pentecostal churches did. Across all denominations, 46% of respondents described their commitment as strong or very strong; 54% described their commitment level as weak. When asked whether the leaders of the various faith communities surveyed had promoted condom use among married members of the faith community within sermons or formal teachings within the six months prior to the assessment, 61% claimed that they had. When analyzed along the lines of denominational affiliation, the survey found that 57% of mainline churches, 54% of Pentecostal churches, and 69% of AICs promoted condom use among married members of their congregations. Across denominational lines, 57% of the respondents described their commitment level to the promotion of condom use among married couples as very strong or strong (30%). Disaggregated, 41% of mainline churches, 59% of Pentecostal churches, and 63% of AICs described their commitment level as strong or very strong. Though the variance between denominations is less pronounced when it comes to the promotion of condom use among married couples as opposed to unmarried partners, the variation remains worth exploring further.

This variation between denominations, in the case of married as well as unmarried couples, is not only striking as an indication of how faith communities in Botswana differ on the issue of condoms, it also shows how faith communities in Botswana seem to differ from faith communities in other parts of sub-Saharan Africa. In Mozambique, for example, Pfeiffer (2002) reports that condoms are never mentioned openly in AICs. However, much of what Pfeiffer reports of practices among AICs in Mozambique – e.g., "sexual fidelity is a constant topic for sermons, group discussions, and consultations with prophets" (Pfeiffer 2002: 184) – holds also for Botswana. Returning to the study by Togarasei et al (2008), when asked whether leadership had openly supported the work of government and other organizations in distributing condoms to people, 42% said that they had. Along denominational lines, again, 39% of mainline and 17% of Pentecostal churches but 59% of AICs said that they supported the work of other sectors to distribute condoms. District-level participatory research workshops revealed that many church leaders believed that there should be a division of labor: whereas faith communities should be encouraged to teach abstinence and fidelity, other sectors should be allowed to promote condom use. Opposition to the condom campaign in Botswana within the faith sector is often more a matter of the manner of promoting condom use rather than of simple distribution: many faith leaders found condom advertisement inappropriate for children and demonstrations on condom use within secondary schools to be offensive. Though most respondents, approximately 80%, said that they encourage open discussion with adolescents about HIV, many suggested that the discussion should take place between children and their parents or a member of the faith community rather than a public health official. AICs (48%) were less likely than mainline churches (83%) to hold sessions for youth dedicated specifically to discussing the risk of HIV. And perhaps the relative success of the condom campaign in Botswana, which has gained acceptance even within many faith communities, is a mixed blessing: some scholars suggest not only that the emphasis on casual or multiple partner reduction rather than condom use accounts for the HIV prevention success that is Uganda (Allen and Heald, 2004; Green, 2003; Epstein 2004, 2005; Shelton, 2004; Hearst and Chen, 2004) but also that "initial antipathy toward condoms might, ironically, have helped promote more fundamental changes in behavior" (Green, et al, 2006: 341). "In Uganda," argues Allen and Heald, "the fact that condoms were not initially introduced"; also "the president's negative attitude towards them, played a part in the social acceptance of sexual behavioral change messages" (2004: 1151).

Though some faith-based organizations are well funded and relatively active in HIV prevention initiatives, abstinence clubs or awareness concerts, many are under-funded and relatively inactive and un-networked. Just as it would be mistaken to treat "traditional healers" in Botswana as a homogenous category, it would be inaccurate to treat all "faith-based organizations" as a homogenous group that speaks with a common voice. Cross-denominational cooperation and collaboration does occur, to a limited degree, under the auspices of several ecumenical associations (e.g., Ministers' Fraternal, BOCAIP). But just as the public health sector and the faith sector are sometimes mutually suspicious, denominations within a shared faith tradition are also sometimes diffident or suspicious of one another. To an outsider, the differences that separate those that constitute the faith sector may seem "minor." Reflecting on the phenomenon of mass aggression, Freud suggests that we should think more carefully about the paradoxical relationship between self-aggrandizement or the over-valuation of oneself, and aggression or the devaluation of others.

Freud discusses the narcissism of minor differences in "The Taboo of Virginity" (1917), "Group Psychology and the Analysis of the Ego" (1922), and "Civilization and its Discontents" (1929). In the earliest essay Freud observes that "it is precisely the minor differences in people who are otherwise alike that form the basis of feelings of strangeness and hostility between them." When it comes to defining the self, Freud believed, what we share in common – e.g., DNA, geography, political history, basic faith creeds, sacred texts – is often less important than the "minor" elements that divide us. Even within the most intimate relationships, within friendship and marriage and relations between parents and children and siblings with one another, "feelings of human kinship compete with emotions of hostility. Rivalries are most intense between neighboring towns, civil wars are the most bitterly fought, and the bitterness of sibling rivalry is as old as Cain and Abel." In his own reflections on Freud's analysis of how "narcissistic self-regard depends on and in turn exacerbates intolerance," Michael Ignatieff claims that "what looks like a minor difference when seen from the outside may feel like a major difference when seen from the inside." Following Freud:

> In the undisguised antipathies and aversion which people feel toward strangers . . . we may recognize the expression of self-love – of narcissism. This self-love works for the preservation of the individual, and behaves as though the occurrence of any divergence from his own particular lines of

development involved a criticism of them and a demand for their alteration (1917: 199).

Following Ignatieff:

> It is precisely because the differences between groups are minor that they must be expressed aggressively. The less substantial the differences between two groups, the more they both struggle to portray those differences as absolute. Moreover, the aggression that is required to hold a group together is not only directed outward at another group, but directed inward at eliminating the differences that distinguish individual from group. Individuals, Freud is saying, pay a psychic price for group belonging (1998: 51).

By extrapolating a bit from both Freud and Ignatieff, it becomes possible to half-understand why faith communities are often hesitant if not occasionally hostile to ecumenical or even cross-denominational cooperation. Faith communities often develop their identities in the very process of articulating their opposition to what an outsider might describe as a nearly identical faith tradition (e.g., between rural Pentecostal Christians and Independent African Churches such as the ZCC): Christians distinguish themselves from Jews and Muslims on the significance of Christ, though both consider most of the Old Testament to be common set of sacred texts or symbols and despite their very similar if not sometimes indistinguishable ethical systems and worldviews. Community-consciousness culminates or crystallizes in the demand for autonomy or self-determination (e.g., Christians from Jews, Protestants from Catholics, the Botswana Lutherans from the South African Lutherans, Pentecostals from non-Pentecostal Christians, and Independent African Churches from missionary denominations). The narrative of oppression and abuses of power is the vector through which minor differences become major – i.e., sufficiently significant or meaningful at least to justify a division within the existing faith community. One's alliance to Christianity, for example, may be demonstrated in one's non-alliance with non-Christian communities of faith or secular organizations; perhaps the justification is that the difference between 'Christian' and 'non-Christian' is by no means minor when it comes to developing one's response to a threat (e.g., a HIV prevention strategy). But perhaps "loyalty" and "group belonging" is not a zero-sum game.

It is inappropriate, however, to apply Freud's analysis of 'the narcissism of minor differences' to the diffidence expressed by some religious communities – including when it comes to intra-sectoral cooperation or collaboration. Freud's notion of personal identity, together with the attending Western assumptions, is fairly far removed from the communitarian ethic espoused in Botswana. When it comes to imagining personal identity in Botswana, the idea is that "I am who I am because of who we are" [*motho ke motho ka batho*] (Gaie and Mmolai: 2004; also Gaie and Jensen: forthcoming, 2010, African Journal of AIDS Research). The social virtues of *botho*, to which VISION 2016 document refers, could be the rhetorical key to a more effective inter-sectoral as well as intra-sectoral HIV prevention campaign. One wonders whether the present public health protections against stigmatization and human rights violations, which some public officials view as "an elaborate rigmarole," would change under the sway of a less Western-based and more *botho*-based approach to preventing HIV transmission as well as the care of PLWHAs.

By collaborating with each other as well as with the public health sector, 'by standing up and joining arms against a common threat' (Togarasei et al, 2008), communities of faith could well play a decisive role in turning the tide on the HIV epidemic in Southern Africa. Faith community leaders in Botswana, from Christians to Muslims and Traditional African Healers, certainly "see and feel" the urgency of the HIV and AIDS crisis; this common heartbeat could well give birth to a collaborative faith-based response: acting together, in heart-smart ways, as if the future depended on us. And indeed it does, "These were all commended for their faith, yet none of them received what had been promised. God had planned something better for us so that only together with us would they be made perfect" (Hebrews 11: 39-40).

In faith, let us say, we believe that God planned something better for us. The lesser plan would allow things to be perfected – or made complete or even improved – without our "*botho*-based" collaborative involvement in our beloved communities (Jensen 2005). And indeed, there is a lengthy and well-intended ecumenical tradition in Botswana (Amanze 2008).

If one believes "in the Jesus of Liberation," to cite one of the DITUMELO 2007 research participants, though this applies to non-Christocentric communities of faith as well, one is committed to working diligently and effectively – to fighting, even – to reducing the causes and conditions of suffering within our respective communities. In Botswana, this means – among other things – working hard to reduce individual risk as well as the social impact of HIV and AIDS. What is the relationship between what we espouse and what we do? Prevention is the optimal defense; at best, faith is both a shield and a weapon for achieving good. Though the head matters, faith is rooted in the good heart, which is also essential to changing behavior. Compassion and faith combine in action. The best prevention campaign would weave existing civil sector values – for example, "*motho ke motho ka batho*" or "*botho*-based" rules of behavior into the public health HIV prevention message; the most effective prevention messages will focus on the many 'merging points' at which faith and knowledge, heart and head, intersect.

The Common Ground: *Motho ke motho ka batho*

Traditional African societies, according to Mawondo (2006: 13), "are widely believed to have been bound by a very strong sense of community". This African sense of persons and communities is captured nicely in Mbiti's dictum, which alludes simultaneously to a family of African proverbs as well as to its European or – more specifically – Cartesian antipodes: "I am because we are and since we are therefore I am." In Setswana, the proverb is *"motho ke motho ka batho"* or *"motho ke motho ka batho ba bangwe"* or in Ikalanga *"nthu, nthu nge(ne) bangwe"*; in Xhosa, *"umuntu ngumuntu ngabantu."* This conception of the self is often considered to be "common to all African languages and traditional cultures" (Shutte 1993: 46); indeed, Mbiti considers this to be "the cardinal point" in the African worldview. For many if not most Africans, and not merely African philosophers, this communal notion of the self is hailed as one of the chief ways in which the African worldview is to be distinguished from the West (Gaie and Jensen, forthcoming, 2010).

Public health programs in developing countries (and among minorities or foreign-born groups within developed countries) would be more effective if those who design and implement programs possessed an empirically based understanding of existing ethnomedical beliefs and practices and designed and implemented programs with these in mind (Airhihenbuwa 1991: 156). This is especially true in the context of public health programs in which compliance with complex treatment regimes or adoption of new behaviors are desirable, as in many contagious or infectious diseases (Green 1999: 217-218).

Taken together, there are significant merging points of intra-sectoral as well as inter-sectoral agreement with respect to HIV prevention programs:

- Both sectors are committed – usually with great passion – to a shared and undeniably good goal: to reducing the risk and impact of HIV and AIDS in Botswana.

- Both sectors are stressing abstinence and fidelity, and many communities of faith are not at all shy about discussing the importance of responsible condom use.
- Both promote, with few exceptions, testing as well as access and adherence to ART.
- Both focus on youth.
- Both stress the importance of psycho-social support systems.
- Both are trying to address the unjust social conditions that contribute to the epidemic.
- Both sectors are working against, in word if not in deed, stigmatization.
- Both are speaking out against alcohol and drug abuse.
- Both are trying, beyond the scope of their prevention programmes, to alleviate the suffering associated with HIV and AIDS by caring for orphans and vulnerable children as well as providing hospice care and counseling.
- Both agree that prevention, especially behavior change education and a more just social system, is the best defense against the ills associated with HIV and AIDS.

These points of consensus suggest common ground for a *botho*-based multi-sectoral and mutually reinforcing, thus more effective, collaboration between faith and public health sectors. By collaborating with each other, as well as with the public health sector, "by standing up and joining arms against a common threat," communities of faith could and should play a more significant if not decisive role in turning the tide on the HIV epidemic in Botswana. Ideally, our HIV prevention campaign in Botswana will increasingly weave faith-based prevention messages into public health HIV and AIDS IEC materials.

Concluding Remarks

Anthropologists, claims Heald (2005: 3), "have not been enlisted into the effort to combat HIV/AIDS in Botswana, nor have they an established position elsewhere." (The same could be said, *a fortiori*, of many other 'academic or scientific sectors'). In view of the *alleged* lack of success of existing interventions, however, perhaps it is not too late for those who design HIV prevention programs to reach out to anthropologists and historians, as well as those studying religion in Africa, many of whom are eager to contribute their "potential insights." The use of "anthropological forms of understanding" and "potential insights" of local practitioners, claims Heald (2003), despite the sustained critique of individualistic intervention strategies (see Farmer, 1999; Manderston and Whiteford, 2000; Seidel, 2003; Waterston, 1997), "have been 'neglected' by those involved in HIV prevention and treatment." But inter-sectoral collaboration is only possible if both sectors are committed to genuine cooperation. In 2005, wrote Heald, the role of anthropologists is "largely a critical one." But it does seem possible, perhaps even essential, that anthropologists or ethnologists and researchers in general – as well as public health officials and members of diverse communities of faith, including "diviners, healers, and churchmen" – change their communitarian role from "largely critical" to decidedly constructive and increasingly collaborative.

Bibliography

Airhihenbuwa, C. *Health and Culture: beyond the Western paradigm.* London: Sage Publications, 1995.
—. "Culturally appropriate AIDS prevention in urban Africa: Implication for health education." *African Urban Quarterly.* Vol. 6:1, 57-59, 1991.
Allen, T. and Heald, S. "HIV/AIDS policy in Africa: what has worked in Uganda and what has failed in Botswana?" *Journal of International Development*, Vol. 16, 2004, 1141–1154.
Amanze, J. N., *A History of the Ecumenical Movement in Africa*, Gaborone: Pula Press, 1999.
—. *Ecumenism in Botswana: The Story of the Botswana Christian Council*, Gaborone: Pula Press, 2006.
Boschman, D. R. *The Conflict between New Religious Movements and the State in the Bechuanaland Protectorate prior to 1949.* Gaborone: University of Botswana, 1978.
Byaruhanga-Akiki, A.B.T. and Kealotswe, O.N.O *Healers and Protective Medicine in Botswana.* Gaborone: University of Botswana, 1995.
Center for Disease Control and Prevention , PEPFAR Botswana country profile. Available from: http://www.pepfar.gov/pepfar/press/81551.htm [Accessed 5 Nov 2006].
Chilisa, B. *The impact of HIV/AIDS on the University of Botswana: developing a comprehensive strategic response,* Gaborone: University of Botswana, 2001.
—. "Educational research within postcolonial Africa: a critique of HIV/AIDS research in Botswana" in *International Journal of Qualitative Studies in Education* Vol. 18:6, 2005, 659 – 684.

Chilisa, B. C., Dube, M. W., Tsheko, N., and Mazile, B. *The Voices and Identities of Botswana's Children: Gender, Sexuality, HIV/AIDS and Life Skills in Education,* Gaborone: UNICEF, 2005.

Cohen, S. Promoting the "B" in ABC: its value and limitations in fostering reproductive health. The Guttmacher Report on Public Policy, 7: October 2004

http://www.guttmacher.org/pubs/tgr/07/4/index.html

Comaroff, J. and Comaroff, J. *Of revelation and revolution.* Chicago: Chicago University Press, 1997.

De Cock, KM, Mbori-Ngacha D, and Marum E. "Shadow on the continent,", www.thelancet.com, Vol. 360, 2002, 68 ff.

De Waal, A. "A disaster with no name: the HIV/AIDS pandemic and the limits of governance," *Learning from HIV/AIDS,* Ellison, G., Parker M. and Campbell, C. (eds.) New York: Cambridge University Press, 2003.

Dube, M. "Adinkra! Four Hearts Joined Together on Becoming Healer-Teachers of African Indigenous Religion/s in HIV&AIDS Prevention," *Journal of Constructive Theology,* Vol. 10:2, 2004, 131-151.

Epstein, H. "The Fidelity Fix," *New York Times Magazine* June 132004.

—. "God and the Fight Against AIDS." *NY Rev of Books,* *52*(7), 2005a. 4/28/05.

—. "God and AIDS (letter response)." *NY Rev of Books,* *52*(9), 2005b, 5/26/05.

Freud, S. 'The Taboo of Virginity,' *Standard Edition,* Hogarth Press, London, 1917, reprint 1953.

Gaie, J. R. B. and Jensen, K. E. "African Communalism and Public Health Policies: On the Importance of Indigenous Concepts of Personal Identity to HIV and AIDS Policies in Botswana" in *African Journal of AIDS Research,* forthcoming, 2010.

Green, Edward C. *Rethinking AIDS Prevention.* Westport, Ct.: Praeger, 2003.

Green, E., Daniel C., Halperin, T., Nantulya, V. and Hogle, J. A. "Uganda's HIV Prevention Success: The Role of Sexual Behavior Change and the National Response" in *AIDS and Behavior,* Vol. 10: 4, 2006, 335-346.

Green, E. *AIDS and STDs in Africa: bridging the gap between traditional healing and modern medicine.* Boulder, Colorado: Westview Press, 1994.

—. *Indigenous Theories of Contagious Disease,* California: Alta Mira Press, 1999.

—. "Traditional Healers and AIDS in Uganda." *The Journal of Alternative and Complementary Medicine* Vol. 6:1, 2000, 1-2.

—. *Indigenous Healers and the African State*, New York: Pact Publications, 1996.

Halperin D.T., Steiner M.J., Cassell M.M., Green E.C., Hearst, N., Kirby D., Gayle, H.D., and Cates W. "The time has come for common ground on preventing sexual transmission of HIV," *Lancet* Vol. 364, 2004, 1913-1915.

Haron, M. and Jensen, K. E. "Religion, identity and public health in Botswana," *African Identities*, Vol. 6:2, 2008, 183 – 198.

Haron, M. et al (Jensen, Mmolai, Nkomazana, Sebina and Togarasei), Ditumelo Secondary Literature Review: HIV Prevention and Faith-based Organizations in Botswana, 2008, see http://hdl.handle.net/10311/368

Heald, S. "Abstain or die: The development of HIV/AIDS policy in Botswana," *Journal of Biosocial Science,* Vol. 38, 2005, 29–41.

—. "An Absence of Anthropology: Critical Reflections on anthropology and AIDS policy and practice in'Africa,'" Ellison, G., Parker, M., and Campbell, C. (eds.) *Learning from HIV/AIDS: a Biosocial approach*, Cambridge: Cambridge University Press, 2003, 210-237.

—. "It's Never as Easy as ABC: Understandings of AIDS in Botswana," *African Journal of AIDS Research* Vol. 1:1, 2002, 1-11.

Hearst, N., and Chen, S. *Condom promotion for AIDS prevention in the developing world: is it working?* Henry Holt & Company, 2004.

Ignatieff, M. "The Warrior's Honor," *Family Planning Studies* Vol. *35*, 1998, 39–47.

Ingstad, B. "The cultural construction of AIDS and its consequences for prevention in Botswana." In *Medical anthropology Quarterly: International Journal for the analysis of health* Vol. 4:1, 1990, 28-40.

Jensen, K. "Personifying the Problem of Evil: The Face of God in an Era of HIV/AIDS" in *Scriptura*, Vol. XV, 2005, 25-31.

Kaleeba, N., Namulondo, J., Kalinki, D., and Williams, G. *Open secret: People facing up to HIV and AIDS in Uganda* (Strategies for Hope Series no. 15). London: ACTIONAID, 2000.

Klausner,R., Wamai, G., Kasonde B., Kawango A., Kagimba, J. and Halperin, D.T. "Is male circumcision as good as the HIV vaccine we've been waiting for?" *Journal of Future Medicine* Vol.2:1, 2008, 11-17.

Landau, P. *The realm of the word: language, gender, and Christianity in a southern African kingdom,* Portsmouth, NH: Heinemann, 1995.

Manderson, L. and Whiteford, L. (eds) *Global Health Policy, Local Realities: The Fallacy of a Level Playing Field,* Lynne Rienner: Boulder, 2000.

Mawondo, S. "Villagers in the City: Reexamining the African Sense of Persons and Community. *BOLESWA Occasional Papers in Theology and Religion,* 2006, 12 – 20.

Mbiti, J. *African Religions and Philosophy.* London: Heinemann, 1969 .

Menkiti, I. "Persons and Community in African Traditional Thought," Wright, R. A. (ed.), *African Philosophy: An Introduction,* Lanham, MD: University Press of America, 1984, 171-182.

Ministry of Health - Botswana *Botswana AIDS Impact Survey* (BIAS 1), 2008.

Nkomazana, F. and Lanner, L. *History of the Church in Botswana,* Pietermaritzburg: Cluster Publications, 2007.

Ntloedibe-Kuswani, G.S.."African Religions and 2001 Population and Housing Census in Botswana." Centre for Continuing Education, University of Botswana, 2003 (http://www.cso.gov.bw/images/stories/Census/paper24.pdf).

Ntseane, P. and Preece, J. Why HIV/AIDS prevention strategies fail in Botswana: considering discourses of sexuality. *Development Southern Africa,* Vol. 22:3, 2005, 347-363.

Petraglia, J. "The Importance of Being Authentic: Persuasion, Narration, and Dialogue in Health Communication and Education" in *Health Communication,* Vol. 24, 2009, 176-185.

Pfeiffer, J. "African independent churches in Mozambique: healing the afflictions of inequality," *Medical Anthropology Quarterly* Vol. 16:2, 2002, 176-99.

Seidel, G. "HIV/AIDS: Behind the rhetoric, whose interests are being served?" *Review of African Political Economy* Vol. 98, 2003, 664–670.

Setiloane, G. *The image of God among the Sotho-Tswana,* Rotterdam: A.A. Balkema, 1976.

Shelton, J. D., Halperin, D., Nantulya, V., Potts, P., Gayle, H., and Holmes, K. "Partner reduction is crucial for balanced "ABC" approach to HIV prevention," *British Medical Journal,* Vol. 328, 2004, 891–893. (http://bmj.bmj journals. com/cgi/content/full/bmj; 328/7444/891)

Shutte, A. *Philosophy for Africa.* Rondebosch, South Africa: University of Cape Town Press, 1993.

Shapiro R. L., Kebaabetswe P, Lockman S, Mogwe S, Mandevu R, Thior I. and Essex, M. "Male circumcision: an acceptable strategy for HIV prevention in Botswana" *Journal of Sexually Transmitted Infections.* Vol. 79, 2003, 214-219.

Stoneburner, R. L., and Low-Beer,D. Is condom use or decrease in sexual partners behind HIV declines in Uganda Presentation, XIIIth International AIDS Conference, 9–14 July, Durban, South Africa, 2000.

Ter Har, G. and Ellis, S. "The Role of Religion in Development: Towards a New Relationship between the European Union and Africa," *The European Journal of Development Research*, Vol.18:.3, 2006, 351–367.

Togarasei, L. "One Bible, many Christianities: the picture of Christianity in Zimbabwe Today," *Zambezia: Journal of humanities of the University of Zimbabwe*, Vol. 32:2, 2006, 20–36.

—. "Cursed be the Past!: Tradition and modernity among modern Pentecostals," *BOLESWA: Journal of Theology, Religion and Philosophy* Vol. 1:2, 2006, 114-132.

Togarasei L., et al. *An Assessment of the Capacity of Faith-Based Organizations for HIV Prevention in Botswana*, Gaborone, Associated Press, 2008.

Trinitapoli and Regnerus"Religion and HIV Risk Behaviors Among Married Men: Initial Results from a Study in Rural Sub-Saharan Africa." *Journal for the Scientific Study of Religion* Vol.45:4, 2007, 505-528.

UNAIDS Epidemic Update, "Male circumcision: Africa's unprecedented opportunity."

UNAIDS (2009). "Epidemic Update," available at http://data.unaids.org/pub/Report/2009/JC1700_Epi_Update_2009_en.pdf

Waterston, A. "Anthropological research and the politics of HIV prevention: towards a critique of policy and priorities in the age of AIDS," *Social Science and Medicine* Vol.44:9, 1997, 1381–1391.

Wilson, D. "Partner reduction and the prevention of HIV/AIDS: the most effective strategies come from communities," *British Medical Journal* Vol. 328, 2004, 848–849.

PART II:

CHRISTIANITY

CHAPTER FOUR

SOME MAINLINE CHURCHES' INVOLVEMENT IN STRATEGIES TO FIGHT HIV AND AIDS IN BOTSWANA

SANA MMOLAI AND JOSEPH GAIE

Introduction

The fight against HIV and AIDS is at different levels, which is necessary given the many factors that are critical in whether or not the battle is won. Whether or not the battle against HIV and AIDS is won is a moral imperative—it is morally required that the battle be won. In other words it would be morally wrong or immoral if HIV and AIDS continued to ravage humanity the way it has and might continue to without human beings trying to stop it. One of the critical things is what ought to be done to stop the disease. The other issue is who ought to do what to stop the disease. It is in this context that different strategies have been employed to fight the disease some of which are the use of condoms, sexual abstinence, faithfulness to one's sexual partner, testing for HIV, care for those infected with HIV, palliation for those suffering from AIDS, cooperation between organizations fighting the disease and embarking upon other courses of action to address HIV and AIDS problems.

All the above strategies have implications for the stakeholders who have to participate in the struggle if something significant is to be achieved. It is important to point out here that when all has been said and done, the critical thing is for the society to engage in ways to intervene and stop the spread of HIV infection. The argument we are making is that for an intervention to succeed the church is an important stakeholder and whatever it does is crucial for the success of any intervention. On the one hand, there is government which has the moral duty to care for the health of the nation. Being a secular state, Botswana's Ministry of Health does not have to be guided by religious sentiments and dogma when it addresses the problems of HIV and AIDS. That has implications because other stakeholders such as the religious community, which is a significant constituency of the government, has to come on board if the efforts of government are to bear fruit. For that to happen there has to be a dialogue or dialogues regarding the matters that touch on the faith of the people. It is clear that faith based organizations and churches are a critical part of the fight against HIV and AIDS (Haron, et al. 2008, Nkomazana 2008, Nkomazana 2008b, L. Togarasei 2008). On the other hand there is concern that some of the strategies that government uses to fight against HIV are contrary to the teachings of some religious communities. The use of condoms, for example, is of concern to many religious traditions and congregations (Togarasei, et al. 2008: 74).

It is therefore expedient that church leadership be considered as part of the stakeholders who can contribute to the fight against HIV and AIDS. So this study looks at some of the strategies that are used by some mainline churches to fight HIV and AIDS and examines how they are taken in by the particular congregations in light of their teachings or beliefs. The important question that the research seeks to answer is how the informants perceive the attitudes of their congregation leaders in relation to the different methods of combating HIV and AIDS. This is important because religious leaders are critical in the faith of many religious people; they are a source of knowledge for the congregation (given that they were trained in some cases for years in matters of the faith) and therefore their opinions count. They are the ones who determine, support, supervise, reinforce and encourage what their followers should believe. It is also important in that we might find that adherents of a religion (in this case congregants) believe or do something that is different from their teachings, in which case we cannot afford to ignore religion as a factor in determining the methods of fighting HIV and AIDS. How membership perceives leadership is also important because it, among other things, reveals whether or not the leadership is synchronistic with the general membership in their attitudes and understanding of the issues discussed. This is particularly true when it comes to matters of sexuality. Helen Jackson (2002: 134) has argued that "sex is said to be the area of human experience most lied about." According to her the influence of religion on behaviour is at the levels of individual and society. At societal level, the strict religious beliefs are accepted and advocated when at the same time at an individual level the same beliefs are often violated. This is relevant to our study because one has to understand the level at which the informants are responding with respect to what they believe about their congregation's leadership. We purposively chose three mainline Christian churches—

Catholic, Methodist and United Congregational Church of Southern Africa (UCCSA) for our study. We used purposive sampling (Best and Kahn 2006: 19) because it is suitable for the purpose of this study. After choosing the said denominations we had to employ convenience sampling (Best and Kahn 2006: 18) of the denominations because they are found in different parts of Botswana. We chose Serowe (Catholic and Methodist); Gaborone (Catholic, Methodist and UCCSA); Kanye (UCCSA); and Pitsane (Methodist). We chose the churches not only for convenience, but also because they are old churches, mostly represented in the study conducted by UB-TRS Ditumelo Research Team (Togarasei et al 2008). These three churches are among the most influential in Botswana, they also have a clear hierarchy that is easy to access and the other two (Catholic and UCCSA) have educational institutions that could help in piloting some HIV and AIDS related interventions.

It is also worth noting that the locations are both in the urban and rural areas, which is important since locality might be an important factor. The study was conducted among 15 participants (2 church leaders, 5 prominent members of HIV and AIDS committees, 2 church secretaries, 6 members of the Women's Fellowship) who are actively involved in HIV and AIDS activities within their churches and denominations.

We collected data by means of in-depth key informant interviews using a standardized interview schedule. We wanted the informants to give us responses to the same questions so that we may compare them to see if there were any differences. For example, what is easy or difficult about leadership in a Catholic parish promoting sexual abstinence may not necessarily be the same for a Methodist one (Best and Kahn 2006: 268).

The above mentioned study conducted by UB-TRS Ditumelo Research Team has established that preaching and encouraging fidelity and abstinence were common strategies among religious organizations. They encouraged condom use mostly but differed about such use by unmarried people. They discouraged stigmatization of people affected and infected by HIV. They provided counseling services and encouraged testing. The major barriers faced by the churches in implementing HIV prevention programmes were lack of resources (facilities, personnel and finance) (Togarasei, et al. 2008: 8-9). The study did not find out what members believed about their leadership regarding the issues that our study investigated such as what they believe is easy or difficult about promoting abstinence and condom use.

Over and above its findings this study discusses the findings of the study conducted by UB-TRS Ditumelo Research Team on condomization, abstinence, testing for HIV, cooperating with other organizations and government on methods of fighting the spread of HIV and AIDS. The current study collected information on what is difficult and easy; what is good and bad; who approves and disapproves the different issues of fighting HIV and AIDS. This is important in that such issues could be dealt with, once identified. For example, the study conducted for Botswana-United States Partnership (BOTUSA) by UB-TRS Ditumelo Team did not ask what was easy and difficult about certain things being done in local congregations such as promoting condom use or sexual abstinence. This study is important in that targeted interventions can be made based on the available information. For example, if a certain parish finds it easy to have leadership promote abstinence until marriage because people are taught as part of their normal catechesis to abstain, then catechesis could be used as an option to promote behaviour change.

Strategies for fighting HIV and AIDS

Sexual abstinence is the most effective method of totally preventing the spread of HIV through sexual intercourse. Unlike methods like condomization that require funds for purchase and distribution of condoms, abstinence does not cost money. It is one of the most practicable—all people are capable of doing it and they do not have to be taught how to do it even though they might have to be told why they have to do it. So from a rational point of view, it is one of the clear options that need close investigation. In addition to the above, it is one of the most controversial methods of preventing HIV. A lot of people agree that it is the safest method but others like Jackson think:

> It is unrealistic to expect the majority of young, healthy, sexually mature males and females to live indefinitely without any sexual release. It is extremely difficult for many men to obey the vow of celibacy throughout their lives and yet the safe release of masturbating is also considered sinful by various religions and cultures. Realistically, if abstinence is advocated, then masturbation should be encouraged to make abstinence easier to maintain over time (Jackson 2002: 120-121).

Osei-Wusu Brempong (Brempong 2007: 80-81) has made the point that abstinence has raised controversy for the church. The controversy is also pointed out by Joseph Gaie and Sana Mmolai (Gaie and Mmolai 2006: 34-35). Sexual abstinence is also mentioned in many instances as a part of the package to fight HIV. It is one of the three ABC (abstain, be faithful and condomise) (Brempong 2007: 80; Nkomazana 2007b; Isaak 2007: 117; Mash 2007: 137ff) methods of HIV prevention.

Condomization is also one of the controversial methods of preventing HIV (Gaie and Mmolai, 2006:35). We note that in the case of abstinence the controversy mainly arises because of the criticisms leveled against the churches for insisting on abstinence even in the face of apparent failure of the method. In the case of condomization, the controversy arises because the church, traditionalists and religious people criticize governments for promoting condoms at the expense of better methods of fighting the disease.

Some people, including church goers, argue that it is not practicable to insist on abstinence alone and to reject condom use altogether. It is reasonable to at least condomize when one is unable to abstain (Jackson 2002: 121; Amanze 2000; Isaak 2007: 113ff). Others argue that the promotion of condoms especially among the youth is likely to increase sexual promiscuity and immorality (Amanze 2000: 207; Kamanga 2007: 108; Akinboboye and Olanipekun 2007: 126; Nkomazana 2007b: 60). It is therefore important to find out further details from our informants regarding this method because then we can design intervention methods that are mindful of their concerns.

Being faithful to one's partner is the least controversial of the three most talked about methods of fighting HIV. Many believers across faiths agree that fidelity is a very highly desirable behaviour. In the context of HIV, it is important to note that fidelity reduces the chances of HIV infection. It is one of the factors that contributed to the reduction level of HIV infection in Uganda where President Museveni is said to have encouraged it and it was known as "zero grazing" (Mash 2007: 137).

It is also important to note that being faithful makes sense when the people concerned are married adults. The unmarried people may be faithful to their current partners but are at risk of infection when they change partners. The state of affairs is most likely for the youth. Rachel Mash has also highlighted the fact that being faithful in marriage does not necessarily guarantee safety for women because they are unable to insist on faithfulness of their husbands—being faithful does not mean one's spouse is faithful. Further, whilst a girlfriend may still be in a position to argue for fidelity and the use of condoms, a faithful wife is not in a position to insist on condom use (Mash 2007: 139).

Testing for HIV is not as controversial as the above. It would appear that many congregations and faith organizations do not have any problems with testing. Many would readily encourage their members to test. It is however important to note that testing can raise many moral problems. For example, is it morally acceptable to force couples who want to marry to test? What about the aspiring priests, can they be tested before their ordination (Akinboboye and Olanipekun 2007, 124-125)? Our study does not investigate these issues but they are important from a moral point of view. If people are prevented from getting married because they are HIV positive; or they are criticized for wanting to have children on account of being HIV positive; or they are denied ordination, is it morally justifiable? These questions are important for our study in that even though it does not investigate them, the ease with which testing is acceptable without any question being raised about the implications of positive results is problematic and therefore needs further investigation.

Palliation and the care for people living with AIDS is very important as a strategy to fight the disease. It is important to find out what is difficult, easy, good or bad about caring in the different congregations. It is almost universally accepted that the people need care. Associated with care are networking by different organizations and congregations. It is important to find out the kinds of issues that arise in relation to these. Thus, challenges faced by different congregations will be important in ensuring that interventions are appropriately carried out.

It is therefore important to have these issues at the back of our minds as we go through the information from our informants since that would be useful in any kind of intervention to address the spread of HIV.

a) Sexual Abstinence

The findings of the study conducted by UB-TRS Ditumelo Team revealed that leadership across most faith communities promotes sexual abstinence (Togarasei et al, 2008). It is also evident from this study that the three selected faith communities lay great emphasis on abstinence in their teachings (UCCSA, 75%; Catholic Church, 83% and Methodist Church, 100%). It is also evident from the findings of the current study that leadership in the selected Catholic, Methodist and UCCSA congregations promote abstinence until marriage because premarital sex is regarded as sin in the Bible. Informants were asked to identify activities carried out in their respective denominations and congregations geared towards the promotion of abstinence until marriage. The following activities were reported:

- Workshops and group discussions
- Teaching during seminars
- Giving health talks to the youth
- Preaching and teaching about abstinence
- Encouragement of sexual abstinence

- Highlighting the bad consequences of failure to abstain

Participants felt that it is good for leadership to promote abstinence before marriage among members of their congregations because religious leaders are more listened to because they are respected by both the congregation and people in general. To this end, it was argued that it is best for people, particularly the congregation to hear such information from the leadership than any other person. It is the feeling of those interviewed that it would be best and good for leadership of every congregation to teach the youth about abstinence before marriage. Some of the reasons given to support the need to promote abstinence among members were:

- It teaches the youth to avoid contracting communicable diseases and HIV and AIDS. Quite a good number of the young people are not yet married and so they become role models
- It helps to prevent various sexually transmitted diseases and HIV and AIDS
- To restore the dignity of children who would otherwise be born out of wedlock

Further, participants felt that the most important factor which makes it easy for the leadership across most Christian churches and congregations to promote abstinence until marriage is the fact that Christian leaders base their teaching about sexual abstinence on the word of God. It was argued that once it is emphasized that it is the will of God to emphasise abstinence before marriage, the congregation would definitely listen and respond positively, unlike when the teaching is based on secular ideas. For instance, in some congregations abstinence is emphasised during catechism classes, pre-marriage lessons and marriage ceremonies.

It has also been highlighted that the promotion of abstinence improves morality, hence the need to emphasise it in most congregations. The other factor raised was that promoting abstinence is also Setswana culture, it is *Botho*. Botho encompasses attempts to help others. "It also applies the case of HIV and AIDS prevention. Botho demands that all be involved in the combat against the disease" (Mmolai, 2007: 71). This being the case, even non-Christians would appreciate its emphasis. However, it has been also highlighted that it is difficult for leadership to promote abstinence among members as illustrated by the following verbatim quotes:

- After we have taught members the benefits of abstinence, they tend to be destructed by many secular ideas, media, etc. For instance, certain movies tempt people to have certain desire to have sex, then it becomes difficult for people to practice abstinence. This becomes the greatest challenge to our efforts in promoting abstinence before marriage among our congregation.
- Not all the youth will abstain; therefore they will end up with unwanted pregnancies. Children can be stubborn. Even when you tell them to abstain, they still want to experience sex
- Some leaders are not faithful though they conduct the teachings about abstinence

Having presented the views on sexual abstinence let us now turn to one of the most controversial methods of fighting HIV.

b) Condomization

According to Togarasei et al (2008) 57% of mainline churches promote condom use among members of their congregations. When analysed along the lines of denominational affiliation the findings of this study reveal that 60% UCCSA, 50% Catholic Church and 80% Methodist Church confirm that leadership has promoted condom use among married members of their congregations. It is, however, evident from the findings of the current study that the majority (75%) of participants from the Catholic Church negate their church's support in promotion of condoms among married couples. One response to the question "has leadership in your congregation promoted condom use among married members of the congregation?" was that: "they advice [couples] to communicate whether they want to use it or not but the church advices them to use the natural family planning; if they choose to use it [condom] the church has no problem with that."

When asked why leadership of some congregations encourages condom use among members, participants explained that discouraging the use of condoms could impede HIV prevention efforts. It is illustrated that once members happen to have unprotected sex with an HIV positive person that would in turn spread HIV. This being the case, most selected congregations seem to be having no choice besides encouraging condom use among their members. Promotion of condom use across churches and denominations is mainly done during counseling of spouses, premarital counseling and health talks.

Further, some participants reported that leadership in the selected churches and denominations support government efforts in supplying condoms to the public in the realisation that condom use prevents the spread of STI's, unplanned pregnancies and reduces HIV infection. Apparently, it is important for some churches to support the government in supplying condoms to the public because faith based communities have realized that HIV spreads at an alarming rate. It has been pointed out that since faith based communities are both affected and infected by HIV, they have to support the government's initiatives in the fight against HIV and AIDS. It is the feeling across most congregations that in supplying condoms, the government has the needs and interests of the future leaders at heart. To this end, it becomes imperative for churches to support the government in distributing condoms to the public to protect the nation from being infected by HIV. It was pointed out that faith communities share the same goal: to protect life.

It appears, however, there is need for faith communities and the government to dialogue on condom use and distribution. This is because it is the view of some churches and denominations that education on condom use should not be made public to young members of the congregations. It was pointed out that even though the youth learn about sex related issues from the media, the majority of them do not fully understand issues related to sexual relationships.   This being the case, denominations should emphasize abstinence among young members of the congregation as this is the principal teaching of Christianity.

The other issue raised was that it becomes difficult for churches to support government initiatives in distributing condoms because their feeling is that condoms should be distributed to adults, not children. It is, however, important to note that while the general population in most churches seem to be supporting government initiatives in distributing condoms, it seems the older generation in some churches is against condom distribution. Participants explained that some churches and denominations are not very keen in supporting the government in condom distribution as this contradicts what faith communities should preach: no sex before marriage and faithfulness within marriage. It was argued that encouraging condom use in a way contradicts what Christian communities should emphasize.

Another aspect which appears to be an impediment for faith communities in supporting the government in condom distribution emanates from the fact that churches and the government seem to be in different platforms about sexuality. Apparently, while the church emphasises abstinence before marriage on the one hand, the government supports condoms and is either tolerant of or silent on the morality of sex outside marriage on the other hand. Furthermore, it is the feeling of most participants that the government does not help faith communities in promoting sexual abstinence hence their reluctance in supporting the government in condom promotion.

It appears most churches have different associations or committees focusing on different issues. For instance, there exist special committees such as Wellness Committees in some congregations, which guide the congregation on what issues to address, as well as spearheading relevant activities. Other congregations have health care personnel responsible for issues related to HIV and AIDS and other diseases. Where there are no such committees, leadership becomes responsible for supporting government efforts in distributing condoms.

The majority of participants from the Catholic Church pointed out that their church does not support the promotion of condom use among married couples as illustrated by these verbatim quotations:

> They have discouraged it

> They do not support supply of condoms because married couples are taught how to take a break (from sex), e.g., when the wife is breastfeeding or if they are staying far from each other

> They feel that people are committing abortion

> May be perceived as promoting promiscuity

> Condom use encourages people to lose morality

> It is against our religion to support condom use

According to most participants, condom use is against the teachings of the Roman Catholic Church. This being the case, the leadership in the selected congregations is perceived as guided by the law of the church to preach against condom use. It is, however, the feeling of 10% of participants from the selected Roman Catholic congregations that faith communities should support government in their efforts to supply condoms to the public because condom use can help in the reduction of diseases, including HIV. It has also been pointed out that social changes, such as the breakdown of family value system and the extended family, the availability of condoms to the youth, the mass media and education, prevalent in Botswana challenge the church to allow condom distribution and utilization.

c) Faithfulness within Marriage

It is evident from Togarasei et al (2008) that most faith communities promote faithfulness within marriage in sermons and teaching, with an overwhelming 96% of mainline churches confirming this activity. When analysed along the lines of denominational affiliation, the results of the study conducted by the Ditumelo Team reveal the overwhelming majority (100%) of UCCSA, Catholic Church and Methodist Church confirming their leaderships' promotion of faithfulness within marriage in sermons.

When asked who approves of the promotion of faithfulness within marriage in sermons, the findings of the current study reveal that in many churches and congregations nobody disapproves of its promotion and in general, leadership (the presiding bishop, minister, deacons, members of the wellness committee, etc) and the entire congregation fully approve of the promotion of faithfulness within marriage among members of the congregation. Promotion of faithfulness within marriage is predominantly done through:

- Workshops and Seminars
- Teaching couples the usefulness of faithfulness
- Bible studies
- Sermons
- Pre and post marital counseling
- Talks
- Encouraging the congregation to be honest

When asked why the faith communities seem to be keen in promoting faithfulness within marriage, it was explained that faithfulness within marriage is considered good because it is capable of building strong marriages. It was further argued that it would enable partners to be faithful and stick to each other. As confirmed, emphasizing faithfulness within marriage has shown good results, as divorces are few and conflicts between couples are also very rare. It is therefore the general feeling within most churches that promoting faithfulness within marriage protects the institution of marriage; enhances trust, love and understanding; reduces the spread of HIV and saves lives of many couples and other parties involved in marriage relationships, as illustrated by these extracts:

> It is good to promote faithfulness among church members. For instance, if I have the HIV and I am faithful to my partner, I would not spread the virus among other people. Being faithful to me would also prevent my wife

from spreading HIV. It is against this background that I argue it is more ideal for the congregation to promote faithfulness in marriage as it has many advantages.

We will become an HIV and AIDS and stress free community

It is central to the teachings of the Christian church

We will not have many divorces, diseases etc. Youth will also learn about the goodness of faithfulness

It is emphasized by the Ten Commandments

Participants further explained that it is easy for most churches and congregations to promote faithfulness within marriage because, like abstinence, the teaching is based on the Bible. From data collected, it is clear that since Christianity emphasises both abstinence and faithfulness, it becomes easy for Christian churches to emphasize these issues. However, promoting faithfulness within marriage has its challenges. In the first place, the difficulty arises from the fact that there is need to hold workshops to teach skills for faithfulness. Such workshops need money and there are times when churches do not have funds. It has also been pointed out that lack of experienced and competent counsellors becomes an impediment to the promotion of faithfulness within marriage. Further, inter-denominational marriages appear to challenge the promotion of faithfulness as some churches do not emphasise faithfulness within marriage. The other difficulty according to one respondent is that "some churches promote the use of contraception." The implication of this concern for inter-denominational marriages lies in the fact that the husband and wife would differ when it comes to the use of contraception. This has the strong possibility of breaking the marriage because couples will be disagreeing on such an important issue.

d) HIV Testing

Besides the ABC campaign, the study conducted by the Ditumelo Research Team sought to find out essential HIV testing activities carried out by faith communities. From the data of this study, 96% of mainline churches promoted testing in sermons (Togarasei et. al 2008). Data from this study further show the majority (100%) of participants from UCCSA, Catholic Church and Methodist Church confirming their leaderships' promotion of HIV testing in sermons and teachings. Data for the current study also reveals that leadership and the entire congregation of most churches and congregations support and promote HIV testing. In general, workshops and visits by HIV and AIDS specialists make it easy for the congregation to participate. Creating awareness among the congregation is also very important.

Further, participants felt that it is important for members of the congregation to know their status because once people know their status, they would be in a better position to take positive actions regarding their lives. It was also mentioned that knowing one's status promotes good health for all. In this way, leadership in most congregations has decided to promote HIV testing among members. The other point raised is that HIV testing enables HIV to be diagnosed and treated early. It was also pointed out that many people get tested in church because there is less stigmatization in the church, a contested view though considering that the church has long been accused of fueling HIV stigma. This being the case, promotion of HIV testing is mainly done through the following approaches:

- Inviting different specialists to the congregation to test various diseases, including HIV.
- Leadership testing first and encouraging others to test.
- Premarital counseling and couples seminars.
- Arranging for HIV testing during church service.
- Putting up notices about testing dates.

However, promotion of HIV testing has its own challenges to these churches. Ignorance within the congregation has been identified as the major challenge. For instance, if the person has not been fully aware of the causes, prevention and consequences of HIV, he or she may fear to test. It also appears that people do not respond to HIV testing campaigns due to different arguments about sexual relationships, contraception and methods to combat HIV and AIDS. Further, combining parents and the young people in meetings and workshops was also identified as another challenge as the combination is capable of impeding freedom of speech among participants. It was suggested that separating parents from the youth during meetings and workshops on HIV and AIDS would be more appropriate and acceptable.

e) Palliation (Supporting People living with HIV and AIDS)

It is evident from the findings of the assessment study conducted by the Ditumelo Team on faith based Organizations' HIV prevention activities that the majority of faith communities support people living with HIV and AIDS through numerous activities. When the results were disaggregated along denominational lines, the survey found that the majority (over 75%) of participants from UCCSA, the Catholic Church and the Methodist Church confirm that their congregations held counseling sessions with, and healing services and prayers for people living with HIV and AIDS (PLWHA). Further, all participants confirmed that their congregations provide direct services to orphans and vulnerable children.

The findings of the current study also reveal that most congregations support PLWHA. The following were verbatim quotes from participants:

- Every year our Committee invites PLWHA to address the congregation about their status and the challenges they face in the community. In our congregation we have also taken the initiative of taking care of more than 300 HIV and AIDS orphans
- We support PLWA by giving out food baskets
- In our church we mainly support PLWHA by visiting them and giving them love
- Those who are infected by HIV are not in any way discriminated by members of the congregation. Furthermore, HIV and AIDS orphans receive various assistance and support from members of the congregation
- Our congregation supports PLWHA by opening centres and donating and giving relevant teaching about HIV and AIDS. Our congregation also supports PLWHA though visitations to hospitals and the sick in the community
- In our congregation members support PLWHA by praying with and tell them not to be afraid; they must be brave
- By opening centres for PLWHA and donating clothes and food to them and by giving relevant teaching about HIV/AIDS
- In my congregation we have a centre for such people and a committee has just been put in office to take care of all health problems, HIV/AIDS included

Since almost all members of various congregations are affected by HIV and AIDS, it becomes easy for churches to support people living with HIV and AIDS. For instance, it is argued by one respondent that:

As I have already said, these are our children, relatives and friends. This being the case, there is no way we can deny them the love and care. We have to bring them closer to us so that they will feel that they are considered as part of the congregation

In general, the leadership (coordinators of various committees within the congregation, ministers, circuit stewards, deacons and other members of the congregation in leadership positions) has realized the need to support PLWHA. This issue has been discussed with congregations and most members accepted the need to do so and decided to take action. Another issue pointed out is that home based care personnel also approve of the congregations' involvement in caring for PLWHA. Apparently, no one in any congregation disapproves of such a noble duty of the church.

f) Networking

Our findings on faith communities networking activities concur with the assessment carried out by the study conducted by Ditumelo Research Team (Togarasei, et al. 2008) that most churches seem to be networking with other organizations, such as, Masiela Trust Fund, Botswana Christian AIDS Intervention Programme (BOCAIP), The Coping Centers for people living with HIV/AIDS (COCEPWA) and other government institutions. From data collected for this study, most participants pointed out that they are prepared to network with other organizations involved in HIV and AIDS activities. One respondent pointed out that "our congregation is willing to work with others to fight HIV/AIDS." Asked why there is a need to network with other churches, one respondent argues that, "...because we have realized that HIV and AIDS affect us all in Botswana. If they are inviting us to network with them, we will be ready to do that as this will enable us to share ideas, etc."

It is also the feeling of the majority of the congregations that networking would assist in minimizing the spread of HIV and AIDS. Churches are also willing to network in order to know what others are doing and learning as "the battle is not ours alone- we need each other." It was emphasised that networking would benefit most churches because different congregations would be are able to share resources, ideas, facilities and materials. For example, it was argued that, "we teach them what we know and experience and they do likewise. We can also share what we have with them."

Besides sharing resources and expertise, networking would assist the churches in attracting more people for testing. For example, combined services where people from different churches and denominations are encouraged to test for HIV and know their status could be more effective than individual churches preaching to their individual congregations. Networking would also improve working relationships among different churches and congregations. Another point emphasised is that, 'Ntwa e *bolotse* (the war has begun), therefore, the congregation acts as advocacy for PLWHA and communities living with AIDS." Apparently, leadership and congregations in most churches approve of church networking. Another issue brought forward was that networking is good because "some churches look up to the Catholic Church." This being the case, networking with the Catholic Church could in a way motivate other churches and denominations to do more for HIV response.

However, it was also pointed out that networking is not a smooth process due to stigma attached to HIV and AIDS. This being the case, people prefer not to be associated with HIV and AIDS related activities. It was also highlighted that the different beliefs and practices within churches and congregations hamper networking for HIV and AIDS actives.

Challenges faced by churches in responding to HIV and AIDS

Data revealed common challenges encountered by most churches and congregations in their fight against HIV and AIDS. It was the general feeling among participants that alcohol and drugs abuse were a serious threat as they explained that unlike in the past, nowadays the majority of the youth take alcohol and use drugs. These intoxicants, it was argued, affect their behaviour and general interpersonal relationships. Some of them who get involved in sexual activities end up having unprotected sex. Proper resources and approaches to dissuade people from alcohol and drug abuse are therefore challenges faced by the churches.

Failure by some denominations to support contraceptives was also identified as a challenge to HIV prevention among some denominations and churches. The fact that certain churches such as the Roman Catholic strongly condemn the use of contraceptives makes it difficult for leadership to accept the distribution of condoms to their members. It was the feeling of some participants that there is need for religious communities to agree on the need to use condoms in this era of HIV and AIDS.

Government's overemphasis of condomization was also identified as a challenge because it is perceived to go against what is arguably the religious communities' effort in promoting abstinence, which is central to the Christian teaching on sexual ethics. However, failure by some denominations to realize that preaching abstinence alone may not help faith communities in winning the war against HIV and AIDS was also identified as a challenge. What can be gathered from this data is that while religious communities wish to emphasise abstinence against the use of condoms, they at the same time realize the need to use condoms as a way of combating HIV and AIDS. The implication of this finding is that perhaps Faith Based Organizations are realising the need to support government's initiatives in promoting condom use among all Batswana.

Lack of financial resources was also identified as a challenge to many HIV prevention strategies and activities. Participants explained that they do not have financial resources to run HIV and AIDS workshops for their respective congregations. It was the feeling of participants that only few churches are aware of available funding which can be utilized for HIV and AIDS workshops and seminars.

Shortage of trained personnel also emerged as a common challenge. It was explained that lack of HIV and AIDS expertise within different congregations impedes HIV prevention initiatives and strategies among religious communities. For example, it was argued that there are times when congregations plan for workshops and find themselves without expertise to resource participants. At times they cancel the workshops, but in most instances they continue without proper expertise. In this way, participants do not fully benefit due to lack of relevant expertise.

Another challenge emphasised by most participants was inadequate knowledge of HIV and AIDS facts. It was explained that some members within the congregations lack basic knowledge of how HIV is transmitted, the difference between HIV and Sexually Transmitted Diseases as well as the difference between HIV and AIDS. This ignorance, it was argued, results in many misconceptions about HIV and AIDS, hence a challenge to HIV prevention initiatives. There is need to first educate church members on HIV and AIDS facts before dealing with HIV prevention strategies. The implication of this finding for the general HIV prevention initiatives is that religious communities need experts within their congregations to address HIV and AIDS facts.

Analysis and Conclusion

Our study has shown that there is a lot that we can learn from the churches' conception of HIV and the methods to deal with it. It is evident that abstinence from sex until marriage coupled with faithfulness to one partner is important in fighting the disease. The difficulty is that insisting on these strategies creates problems. For instance, there are differences in the way the church addresses abstinence thereby making it possible for confusion and lack of cooperation.

Our research has confirmed that there are differences in understanding abstinence as a method of fighting HIV infection. This means any intervention attempt has to take cognizance of the fact that ideas about the role of abstinence are divergent. The faith community does not necessarily mean exactly the same thing when they talk about abstinence. We have also learned that there are certain things that are difficult about promoting abstinence for the church because as expressed by one of the informants "the difficult part is when it is said during Mass where there are young and old, our culture or tradition take talking about sex to young children (10-14) as taboo. It is taboo to do so." This is confirmed by the literature for example (Ouko 2007: 87-88). One difficulty that arises for the church is the fact that people behave differently from what they believe so that even if the church teaches abstinence it does not necessarily follow that the members will be abstinent. Research has shown this as well (Zamberia and Gathu 2006) so there is need to assess the relationship between belief and behaviour.

The major difficulty with the church as regards condom use is that it seems to contradict what the church teaches, namely abstinence in the case of unmarried couples. It also raises fears of the church promoting immorality and sexual permissiveness or promiscuity. The difficulty in supporting government to distribute condoms is that whilst it wants to supply all sexually active people, the church would rather supply only a section of that population. Sometimes it is not easy to do that. For instance, if the head of the church disapproves of their members helping the government to supply condoms then it is not going to be easy for the members to freely participate in matters pertaining to condom use and distribution.

Generally, there is nothing bad about promoting faithfulness in marriage according to our informants but it is important though to note that the promotion of faithfulness in marriage poses danger for faithful partners if the other partner are unfaithful. So, more needs to be explored in terms of the dangers posed. It is also important to note that faithfulness is important from a moral point of view since its practice is consistent with good behaviour. So its promotion in itself is not a bad thing at all.

People generally will promote testing as our data suggests, but it is important to note that an HIV positive result could have undesirable consequences for the subject since they face discrimination and other kinds of stigmatization. If an HIV positive person wants to get married there is going to be moral debates about their rights in marriage and so on. The issue of whether they have the right to have sex with their HIV negative partner and so on would need to be addressed. In actual fact the

Catholic Church, for example, faces a problem in that it requires the inclusion of having children and the consummation of marriage as being essential in determining its validity. This means if a discordant couple tries to marry without intending to have children or do not have sex without a condom to consummate the marriage then there could be problems of validity for the marriage (Leshota 2007). These are the issues that need to be investigated further by conducting further research in other denominations and churches.

It is clear that many congregations appreciate the need to cooperate with other faith organizations to tackle the disease. There is a lot of good for that but on the other hand the concepts and ideas that inform the believers are important in determining the extent to which this cooperation can take place. So, further research is needed to derive maximum benefit from the willingness by churches to cooperate.

The willingness by many congregations to support people living with HIV and AIDS is important because stigma can be defeated. But it is also important to further discover the other problems that people living with the disease and those who ought to help them face in the process.

Theological differences, misapplication, and misunderstanding of theological issues can possibly be the most challenging problems that believers have to face in addressing the problem. This is because if somebody believes God has given a directive it requires a lot of convincing and research for the person to believe otherwise. Challenges of resources are easier to address than theological arguments.

From the above we can conclude that indeed the churches are involved in attempts to fight HIV infection. They are, however, not freely doing so because of a number of issues that they raised. The conflict with the government on condomization and abstinence is one of the issues. Some practices of some denominations are also part of the problem including lack of resources both personnel and financial. The informants do give the impression that there is need to go beyond the denominations and church practice if the scourge is to be overcome. The information gathered suggests the critical importance of the church in any intervention strategies to fight the disease.

Bibliography

Akinboboye, O. and Olanipekun, T. O. "HIV/AIDS and Christian Ethics in Nigeria." in Amanze J.N., Nkomazana F. and Kealotswe O.N. (eds) *Christian Ethics and HIV/AIDS in Africa*, Gaborone: Bay Publishing, 2007, 119-141.

Amanze, J.N. "Covenant with Death: the attitude of the churches in Botswana towards the use of condoms by Christians, and its social implications." *Botswana Notes and Records* 32, 2000, 201-208.

Best, J. W. and Kahn, J. V. *Research in Education.* 10. Boston & Cape Town: Pearson Education Inc., 2006.

Brempong, O. "HIV/AIDS in Africa: Christian Ethics in Ghana." in Amanze J.N., Nkomazana F. and Kealotswe O.N. (eds) *Christian Ethics and HIV/AIDS in Africa*,. Gaborone: Bay Publishing, 2007, 70-85.

Gaie, J. and Mmolai, S. "Condomization as a Method to fight HIV and AIDS: Implications fo" Botho." *BOLESWA Journal of Theology, Religion and Philsophy, Vol* 1:2, 2006, 28-47.

Haron, M., Jensen, K., Mmolai, S., Nkomazana, F., Sebina, L. and Togarasei, L"Ditumelo Secondary Literature Review: HIV prevention and faith-based organizations in B"tswana." *BOLESWA Journal of Theology, Religion and Philosophy Vol* 2:1, 2008, 1-64.

Isaak, P. J. "Social Ethics, and HIV/AIDS in "amibia." Chap. 9 in *Christian Ethics and HIV/AIDS in Africa*, in Amanze J.N., Nkomazana F. and Kealotswe O.N. (eds) *Christian Ethics and HIV/AIDS in Africa*,. Gaborone: Bay Publishing, 2007, 111-118.

Jackson, H. *AIDS AFRICA Continent in Crisis.* Harare: SAFAIDS, Sida, UNESCO, UNFPA, 2002.

Kamanga,M. "Christian Ethics and HIV/AIDS in Africa with Reference to"Malawi." In Amanze J.N., Nkomazana F. and Kealotswe O.N. (eds) *Christian Ethics and HIV/AIDS in Africa*,. Gaborone: Bay Publishing, 2007, 105-110.

Leshota, P. L. "Problematization of the Catholic Church's Understanding of Marriage within the Context of HIV&AIDS," *BOLESWA Journal of Theology, Religion and Philosophy* Vol 1:3, 2007, 37-56.

Mash, R. "Christian Ethics and HIV/AIDS in South Africa: Sex Education in the Anglican"Church." In Amanze J.N., Nkomazana F. and Kealotswe O.N. (eds), (2007).*Christian Ethics and HIV/AIDS in Africa*, Gaborone: Bay Publishing, 2007, 129-141.

Nkomazana, F. "Elias K. Bongmba (2007), Facing a Pandemic: The African and the Crisis of AIDS, Waco Texas: Baylor University Press, 251 pages, notes, Works Cites, Index, ISBN: 1-"32792-1" *BOLESWA Journal of Theology, Religion and Philosophy (BJTRP)*, 2008, 161-162.

—. "The book AIDS and you by Dr Patrick Dixon." *BOLESWA Journal of Theology, Religion and Philosophy (BJTRP)*, 2008, 159-161.

—. "Christain Ethics and HIV/AIDS in Botswana," in Amanze J.N., Nkomazana F. and Kealotswe O.N. (eds) *Christian Ethics and HIV/AIDS in Africa*, Gaborone: Bay Publishing, 2007, 48-69.

Ouko, E. "Christian Ethics and HIV/AIDS in Kenya." in Amanze J.N., Nkomazana F. and Kealotswe O.N. (eds) *Christian Ethics and HIV/AIDS in Africa,*. Gaborone: Bay Publishing, 2007, 86-92.

Togarasei, L, Haron, M., Jensen, K. E., Mmolai, S., Nkomazana, F., and Sebina, L. *An Assessment of the Capacity of Faith-Based Organizations for HIV Prevention in Botswana.* Gaborone: Associated Press, 2008.

Togarasei, L. "Ezra Chitando, Living with Hope: African Churches and HIV/AIDS I, Geneva: World Council of Churches Publication", 2007." *BOLESWA Journal of Theology, Religion and Philosophy (BJTRP)*, 2008, 162-164.

Zamberia, A. M. and Kamanja, G. "The Role of Religious Faith in HIV and AIDS Prevention: The case of the University of Swaziland."*BOLESWA Journal of Theology, Religion and Philosophy*, Vol. 1:2, 2006, 1-27.

CHAPTER FIVE

HEALING IN THE AFRICAN INDEPENDENT CHURCHES IN THE ERA OF HIV AND AIDS

OBED KEALOTSWE

Introduction

This chapter discusses healing in the African Independent Churches (AICS), in the era of HIV and AIDS. The chapter argues that the AICS have always played a great role in the healing of various diseases and ailments even before the advent of HIV and AIDS. Many researches, that have been done in the history, theology and nature of the AICS have shown that the AICS are primarily healing churches. Such researches, to mention a few, include those of West (1975), Daneel (1987), Amanze (1998) and Kealotswe (1987). In most cases, their healing methods and the medicines they use are based on faith. The medicines which are used, which are known as *sewacho* (singular) and *diwacho* (plural) do not necessarily heal on themselves. They heal when the patient has faith. It is for this reason that this chapter tries to examine the healing methods and the concepts of healing in the AICS in the era of HIV and AIDS. The chapter starts by defining the AICS, with special reference to Botswana. It then briefly discusses the healing methods of the AICS, which have been blamed for the spread of HIV and AIDS in Botswana. The chapter will then show any changes that have taken place in the healing activities of the AICS since the outbreak of HIV and AIDS. The changes, include whether the methods used are static or they move with time in consideration of health risks involved in healing.

Who are the African Independent Churches?

The study of the AICS has been made by several people since their beginning in Africa towards the end of the nineteenth century. In South

Africa, a study was made by Sundkler (1961), in the rest of Africa by Barrett (1968), in West Africa by Turner (1967) and in Zimbabwe by Daneel (1971). In Botswana, works on the general lives of the AICS and their healing practices have been done by Kealotswe (1987) and Amanze (1998). These authors have identified two kinds of AICS. First, are the independent churches. The Independent churches are the new religious movements which broke away from the missionary founded churches for two main reasons. The first reason was the failure of missionary Christianity to recognize some aspects of African traditional religious beliefs and practices. These churches constitute the bulk of the Zionist churches. The second category is that of the indigenous movements. These movements were spontaneous uprisings against Christianity and the white people. Most of them have been influenced by Christianity but they do not see themselves as Christians. Examples are those of the Mumbo cult in Kenya (Barrett 1968), and Donna Beatrice (Daneel, 1978) in the Congo. In Botswana, the most known of these movements is the Guta Ra Mwari (Amanze, 1994).These movements had some Christian elements but they were basically revolt movements against the white people and their Christianity. Although many researchers have used the terms indigenous and independent interchangeably, this does not reflect the true situation on the ground as believed by the movements themselves.

From the Zionist movement came other two distinct movements. These were, according to Sundkler (1961 and 1976), the Ethiopians and the Apostolics. The Ethiopians were formed by some educated Africans who wanted to be given recognition and administrative powers in the church. Failure by the missionaries to grant them power, made them to break away and form the Ethiopian Churches (Sundkler, 1961), based on Psalm 68:31, "Ethiopia shall stretch out her hand to God." To the Ethiopian church leaders, this meant a unified church independent of missionary control. The Apostolics are also a later development which did not support any inclusion of African traditional religious beliefs and practices in their faith. They claim to follow the tradition of the Apostles of Jesus and use only pure water in their healing activities.

With reference to Botswana, a study of AICS was made by Amanze (1994) resulting in an anthology. Kealotswe (1987, 1993, and 1994) has made a focused study on the Head Mountain of God Apostolic Church in Zion (HMG). The above studies basically show three types of AICS in Botswana. These are the Independent Churches, Indigenous Movements and the Apostolics. These divisions or classifications, are not clear because there is a lot of mixing up of the traditions of the churches. This is caused by the commercialization of healing which makes the different movements to compete and in the process, copying ideas from others, which are not part of their history. The distinctions remain in doctrinal emphasis where one movement will distinguish itself from others by prescribing different ways of baptizing people, having the Holy Communion in a different fashion or some special church uniforms.

When it comes to healing, there is an aspect of the AICS which one has to understand. Many studies on the AICS have shown that there are AICS which have integrated many African Traditional Religious beliefs and practices in their Christianities. Amanze (1998) and Kealotswe (2005) have come across cases whereby, a traditional healer's clinic has both the traditional divination bones (*Ditaola)* and the Bible, which are both used for diagnosing the patient. Many researchers have realized this integration but they had never been any clear explanation about this situation until recently. In my latest interviews with Traditional Healer Practitioner (THP), Chidoda (2008), he gave an explanation of this phenomenon. According to THP Chidoda, when a person is called into prophecy, there are two basic things which take place in the life of the person. This, according to Chidoda, has led to the emergence of two categories of healers. Thus there are two categories of traditional healers according to him. The first category is that of a person who is possessed by an ancestral spirit. Such a person becomes ill and sometimes gets mentally deranged. The person could be prayed for and get the ancestral spirit exorcised (Pudiephatswa, 2001, Chidoda, 2008). The person then becomes a prophet and is believed to be possessed by the spirit of Jesus Christ. The second category is that of a person who still, is possessed by an ancestral spirit. Such a person sees visions and can diagnose people of various ailments, and diseases. Since such a person is a member of the church, the person is prayed for so that the spirit of Jesus Christ should overcome that of the ancestor. Such a person is taken to the baptismal pool to be cleansed of the ancestral spirit through seven immersions in the water. When the prophets go to the baptismal pool, the ancestral spirit will appear in the form of a water snake, which will just emerge from the bush and runs into the water. If the prophets pray for that water and ritually wash the possessed person in it, that person will have two gifts. The person will have the gifts of prophecy both from the ancestors and also from Jesus Christ. This is the type of prophet who integrates the two forms of healing. If the prophets fear the snake and postpone the washing to another time when the snake does not appear, that person will be exorcised of the ancestral spirit and become a prophet using only the spirit of Christ.

It is, however, very difficult for an ordinary observer to make any distinctions between these two kinds of prophets. The problem is that, in spite of the fact that the prophet who claims to use the spirit of Christ despises the ancestral spirit, one cannot tell the difference when it comes to the healing methods. The two types of prophets basically use the same methods. On the other hand, the Apostolics claim to use only holy water. The indigenous movements have their own sources, which are determined by their leader. These are the complications which one should have in mind when discussing the healing practices of the AICS.

Healing in the African Independent Churches

The issue of healing features in all the researches that have been done on the AICS. Most of these researches (Byaruhanga-Akiki and Kealotswe, 1995, Amanze, 1998) identified some dangerous tools which are used by the AICS when they attend to their patients. The most common tool which was not conducive to health has been the use of *sepeiti* (enema). In many cases, it has been observed that, when enema was applied to patients, the nurse *(mmamosebeletsi)* would use the same syringe on many patients. This could either be a syringe or a jug with a long tube which is inserted into the anus of the patient. Water mixed with various medicines, commonly referred to as *sewacho* (singular) or *diwacho* (plural), would be pumped into the anus of the patient. After a few minutes, the patient would have his or her stomach running. The process is carried on for a number of days depending on the nature of the disease. It is believed that the water which is pumped into the stomach cleanses the stomach and the bowels. In the process, it also cleanses the blood of the patient. Contrary to biological evidence, African traditional healing and that of the AICS, does not separate the blood vessels from all the other organs of the body. All diseases which are in the patient's body are expelled. The problem with the use of one syringe is that it is easy to transmit diseases from some patients to others. This method is unacceptable in the era of HIV and AIDS.

The second criticized method is that of using the same razor blades when cutting patients to remove blood for various treatments. This method is common with the Zion Christian Church (ZCC). The method is not good in the era of HIV and AIDS because the HIV could be easily transmitted to other patients once the blood from an infected person, which remains in the razor blade, finds its way into the blood of the other patient. These two methods caused a lot of complaints on the healing methods of the AICS when HIV and AIDS broke out in Botswana in around 1985 (Kealotswe 2007:14-27). Numerous radio broadcasts, workshops with traditional healers and church healers were conducted all over the country to conscientize people against the use of healing methods which could spread the HIV. By the year 2000, church healers and traditional healers were conscientized about HIV and AIDS and were asked to stop practices which could spread the HIV. Many churches refrained from using the same utensils on many patients. Today such healing practices are rarely practiced.

The concept of HIV and AIDS and its healing by the AICS in Botswana

It is important to understand that healing in the AICS is holistic. The concept of disease is holistic in that a disease is understood to be caused by many factors. The first cause of disease is the poor relationship between the individual person, the family, the relatives, the society in general, the environment or nature, the ancestors (*badimo,* and finally God (*Modimo).* The interaction between all these factors causes good health or disease, depending on whether the relations are good or bad. This philosophy behind health and healing raises questions in the healing practices of the AICS. The questions are those of identity. It becomes difficult to classify the healer-prophet, as to whether he or she integrates the healing practices or claims not to integrate them. HIV and AIDS is believed by many AICS to be an accumulation of many diseases. Some of the diseases could have been caused by the violation of taboos or by the curse of the ancestors. To the integrating healer, there is nothing wrong in telling the patient that the disease is caused by failure to obey the demands of an ancestor. To the prophet who claims to use the spirit of Christ, the explanation to the patient could be that the angel (*ingilozi* or *moengele*) could be unhappy about something and let disease strike the patient. These explanations are not in any way different. The healing methods of the two types of healers are in all aspects the same. The examples given below will illustrate the problems.

It has been stated above that the concept of disease as understood by the AICS is holistic. To give some examples and the treatment of HIV and AIDS, let us briefly focus on HIV and AIDS and women. AICS believe that HIV and AIDS, especially in women, is caused by the accumulation of different venereal diseases in the womb of a woman. which then become incurable. The accumulation of diseases in the womb of a woman is caused by having many sexual partners. In traditional Botswana customs, a woman is not allowed to have sexual intercourse with several men because she will develop an incurable disease due to the accumulation of different sperms in her womb. To cure this disease, which is now understood to be HIV and AIDS, Prophetess Noga (Gaborone, 2000), stated that the disease is generally referred to as *popelo*, the womb. When women, especially girls, come to her complaining about *popelo*, she first of all massages the womb by applying some Vaseline petroleum jelly on the stomach and then pressing the parts of the stomach where the womb is located. This continuous process, which might take three or more days, will soften the womb and make the sores in the womb to be crushed so that either blood or some water begins to come out of her womb. When this process begins, she then mixes some water with salt and some specific *diwacho*, which she did not want me to know. She then takes a syringe and pumps some water into the womb. After some few minutes, she inserts the syringe again and removes all the dirt from the womb. Several undertakings of this method, which might take some weeks or a few days, remove all the diseases from the womb of the woman. The salt, which is included in *diwacho*, dries up the wounds in the womb whilst other *diwacho* heal the wounds. This same method is used for healing the womb when a woman or a girl has committed abortion.

AICS also treat diarrhea, which is generally thought to be a sign of HIV and AIDS. When a woman or a man has a constantly running stomach, that is interpreted as a symptom of HIV and AIDS infection. According to Prophetess Noga, when she gets such a patient, she mixes some *diwacho* and some salt with large amounts of water, approximately ten litres. In spite of the fact that the patient has already lost a lot of water due to dehydration, Prophetess Noga will still use *sepeiti,* enema to cleanse her patient. This could appear detrimental to the eyes of Western medical practitioners but to the AICS, that is a different concept. According to Prophetess Noga, the water that is pumped into the patient through the anus, is meant to cleanse the bowels and the intestines. The water is pumped into the patient. After a few minutes the patient goes to the toilet and emits all the water. The patient comes back again and more water is pumped into the stomach through the anus. The process goes on until the ten litres of water is finished. The belief is that, whilst some of the water comes out, some of it is medicinal and heals the wounds which are in the bowels and intestines. The salt dries up the wounds whilst other herbs force the wounds to move out of the stomach and appear outside for easy healing. The wounds which are on the body are easily treated by smearing with some Vaseline mixed with some *diwacho*. The general belief in the AICS' healing practice, which is similar to that of traditional healers, is that for a disease to be cured, it must be forced out of the stomach. Thus, the draining of the stomach is a way of taking the disease out of the stomach. A few days of this process makes the patient to be better. If the patient could not eat, he or she would start eating. The patient starts by drinking some milk, then porridge and finally solid food. After some days, weeks or months, the patient claims to have been healed of HIV and AIDS.

In the case of a male patient, HIV and AIDS is sometimes thought to be a result having the urinary system blocked by venereal diseases. Prophetess Noga said in such cases she mixes some *diwacho* with water and some salt. She gives the patient to drink the mixture. After some minutes, the patient will start urinating. The urine will be mixed with pus and sometimes blood. The patient is also given some *sepeiti* (enema) by a male prophet, with the prescription done by Prophetess Noga. The ten litres of water which is pumped into the stomach of the patient drains out all the dirt from the stomach. At the same time, the amount of water, which could be five litres, which the patient drinks forces the patient to urinate regularly. It is believed that the cleansing of the bowels, together with the cleansing of the bladder and the urinary system makes the patient to feel much better. In case the urine does not come out, Prophetess Noga advises the male prophet and guides him on how to wear a glove and insert his finger into the anus of the patient. The prophet will press on some glands leading to the scrotum. In the process, the patient's penis gets erect and ejaculates all the dirt from the bladder. After some period of treatment, ranging from one week to several weeks, sores will develop on the abdomen and sometimes on the glands of the penis. The belief is that these sores were inside the body and they are forced out in order to be healed easily. Some Vaseline mixed with some *diwacho* is then smeared on the patient and the wounds heal. The patient then believes that he is healed of HIV and AIDS.

The above healing practices are common amongst all the Zionist churches. The Apostolics generally claim to use some holy water and prayer in healing their patients. One example is that of the Lambs' Followers Church, in Maun, which was founded and is led by Morongwa, the Messenger (Kealotswe 2001). In this church, most of the patients are diagnosed by Morongwa, in the presence of a *mosebeletsi* (nurse) or some prophet. Morongwa makes the prescriptions while the *mosebeletsi* writes everything in a book, so that he or she cannot forget what had been explained by Morongwa. The following are examples of prescriptions to patients. Their names have been withdrawn for ethical reasons.

Sunday 14 February 1999
Tlhatlhobo
1. Thuso
*nwa metsi a sejeso a le bothitho 7 days.
*metsi a pelo le madi a le tsididi 7 days.
*metsi a meleko 7 days go tlhapa .
*karametso 3 days o tlodisa 2 days.
*kgatiso 4 days o tlodisa 1 day.
*tshidilo 6 days o tlodisa 1 day.
*sepeiti 3 days o tlodisa 1 week.

Translation
- drink some hot water for treating food-poisoning for seven days.
- drink some cold water for treating the heart for seven days.
- wash in fortification water for seven days.
- fumigation for three days, omitting two days in between the treatment.
- pressings for four days omitting one day in between the treatment.
- massage for six days omitting one day in between the treatment
- enema for three days with intervals of one week in between the treatment.

2. Thuso
*nwa metsi a a bothitho a madi.
*tlhapa ka metsi a meleko 2 weeks.
*kgatshiwa ka metsi a meleko 3 days o tlhomaganya.
*tshidilo ka metsi 5 days o tlodisa 2 days.

Translation
- drink hot water for healing the blood
- wash in fortification water for two weeks.
- splash with fortification water for three successive days.
- massage using water for five days omitting two days in between the treatment.

3. Thuso
*nwa metsi a madi a le tsididi.
*tlhapa ka metsi a meleko 3 weeks.
*karametso ya senyama 7 days.

Translation
- drink cold water for healing the blood
- wash with fortification water for three weeks
- fumigate using water for bad luck for seven days

4. Thuso
*go nwa general e e bololo.
*go nwa general e le tsididi.
*tshidilo 4 days o tlodisa 2 days.
*8 months tshidilo 5 days o tlodisa 2 days.
*sepeiti kgwedi e fela.
*tlhapa ka metsi a meleko.

Translation
- drink mild general water
- drink cold general water
- massage for four days omitting two days in between
- 8 months of massage done successively for five days omitting two days in between
- enema at month end
- wash with fortification water.

5. Thuso
*nwa metsi a dintho.
*tlhapa ka metsi a bana 5 days.
*tshidilo ka metsi 4 days a tlodisa 1 day.
*go tabiwa 3 days.

Translation
- drink water for sores
- wash with children's water for five days.
- massage with water for four days omitting a day in between.
- to be fortified for three days.

6. Thuso
*nwa metsi a popelo a le bololo.
*nwa metsi a dintho a le bothitho.
*nwa metsi a pelo le madi a le tsididi.
*karametso ya bomme 3 days o tlodisa 2 days o kgatshiwa.
*tsidilo 4 days o tlodisa 1 day.
*sepeiti 1 day.

Translation

- drink warm water for the uterus
- drink hot water for curing sores
- drink cold water for the heart and blood
- fumigation for women for three days omitting two days in which one is sprinkled with water
- massage for four days omitting one day
- enema for one day.

The above cases are typical Apostolic. The patients are given water which has been blessed by the Prophet or Bishop. In spite of the fact that some of the water could be prayed for in advance, for the healing of some common diseases and ailments, the healers state strictly that they never use any *diwacho* like the Zionist churches. The above examples are used in various combinations for the healing of People Living With HIV and AIDS (PLWHA). In 2004, I visited the *diagelo* of Morongwa in Maun. *Diagelo* is like a Primary Hospital where many AICS keep their patients for healing (Kealotswe 2002). When they fail to heal them, they refer them to Government or private hospitals. There were more than ten patients who were housed in the different rooms. Most of the patients were PLWHA under home-based care. Morongwa had made some prescriptions for them. Some of the patients told me that they were feeling much better because they could eat some food, which they were not able to do when they were at Maun Hospital.

The other common example of a disease which is associated with HIV and AIDS is *Boswagadi*. *Boswagadi* comes from the word bereavement in Setswana and other Botswana languages. The religious tradition and custom is that a woman who loses a husband through death, should undergo some ritual healing before she could have sex with another man. Many Botswana cultures do not have sexual taboos for men because, even in normal life, before death, a man is allowed by almost all Botswana cultures to have sex with any other woman, besides his wife, provided, in doing so, he does not violate another man's rights over the woman. For this reason, *Boswagadi* is more associated with women than men. Different peoples of Botswana treat *Boswagadi* in different ways. The AICS, however, have an almost common way of treating *Boswagadi*. The disease, *Boswagadi*, affects both men and women. The major symptom of the disease is the swelling of body limbs, especially the ankles, and other joints of the body. The second symbol is a continuous cough which does not get healed. This cough is referred to as *thibamo*, which translates tuberculosis in Western concepts. The patient also loses weight and becomes lean. It is for this reason that when HIV and AIDS started in Botswana, it was simply referred to as *Boswagadi,* due to similar symptoms.

The healing of *Boswagadi*, which is still believed by many healers now to be the healing of HIV and AIDS, takes the following form: When the patient comes to the healer- prophet, the first treatment is that of massaging with some Vaseline. The massage is meant to loosen the stiff swollen joints so that the patient could move the body. This is followed by enema, *sepeiti*, because in many cases, the stomach of the patient will be swollen and the patient might not even be able to eat any food. The enema will remove most of the dirt that had accumulated in the stomach because the *diwacho* that are used also have some nutrients in them. Once the patient starts to eat and be able to move the body, fumigation is done. This is the process in which some *diwacho* are put into boiling water into which some hot stones are also added. The patient is carefully lowered above the container of the hot water, covered with a blanket and forced to inhale the hot steam from the water. In the process, the patient vomits water mixed with foam. The foam is believed to be coming out of the lungs which it had blocked causing *thibamo*. In the process, the lungs open up and the patient breathes normally. The treatment might take some days, weeks or even months, but finally, many patients have claimed to have been healed. This healing method is done by almost all the Zionist Churches with slight variations. It is also done by the traditional healers with some little variations. The problem, which this chapter addresses, is as to whether the healing practices outlined above could be called the healing of HIV and AIDS.

General Assessment of the above healing methods

It is a very difficult task to make an evaluation of the above healing methods and state categorically whether they are false or true. The problem arises due to two major observations. The first one is that in Botswana cultures, there is no concept of an incurable disease. What remains incurable is a disease resulting from a curse. Once the demands of the ancestor or any person who had made the curse are met, the patient gets healed. Many church prophets and traditional healers believe that they can help patients to appease their ancestors if they are suffering from a disease that is associated with some curse. *Boswagadi* is more of a violation of taboos and rituals rather than a curse. It is therefore, healed without some reference to the ancestors.

The second problem is that many people who go to AIC prophets do so on faith. Once they have the faith that they will be healed, they miraculously get healed, probably not necessarily by the medication but through their faith. It is then very difficult to make any objective assessment of such healings.

Looking at the healings, from a scientific point of view, there are some elements of truth in the healings. What remains true is the fact that some opportunistic diseases which attack people with HIV are healed by the AICS. There is all scientific evidence that a person cannot live without eating any food. The first success of the AICS in healing HIV and AIDS patients is that they clean the stomach, bowels and intestines of a patient. By destroying the wounds which were in the stomach and improving the appetite of the patient, the AICS make the patient eat and develop some energy. The treatment then, works similarly to anti-retroviral drugs (ARVs), which keep PLWHA alive for years. In my researches, I have come across many people who claim to have been healed of HIV and AIDS. Very few do understand that they might still have the virus, which is kept low by the treatment they get from the AICS.

As a way forward, my research findings and the evidence from many people who are HIV positive but are alive because of the treatment they receive from the AICS, it is important that the healings of the AICS should be given some serious consideration in the fight against HIV and AIDS in Botswana.

Conclusion

The AICS play a significant role in attending to HIV and AIDS patients. Even if their healing could only be by faith induced by placebos, they play a significant role in the fight against HIV and AIDS. Secondly, many AIC leaders have adopted healing methods which do consider the fact of the existence and possible spread of HIV and AIDS. They then use safe methods in order to avoid those which could spread HIV and AIDS.

Bibliography

Amanze, J. N. *Botswana Handbook of Churches*, Gaborone: Pula Press, 1994.
—. *African Christianity in Botswana: The case of the African Independent Churches,* Gweru: Mambo Press, 1998.
Barrett, D. *Schism and Renewal in Africa*, Nairobi: Oxford University Press, 1968.
Byaruhanga-Akiiki and Kealotswe, O. *African Theology of Healing,* Gaborone: Printworld (PTY)Ltd, 1995.

Daneel, M. *Old and New in Southern Shona Independent Churches, Volume 1: Background and Rise of the Major Movements,* The Hague: Mouton, 1971.

Kealotswe, O.N. *Healing in the African Christian Churches,* Bochum: Ecumenical; Scholarship Program, 1987.

—. *Doctrine and Ritual in an African Independent Church,* Unpublished PHD Thesis, University of Edinburgh, 1993.

—. *An African Independent Church leader: Bishop Smart Mthembu of The Head Mountain of God Apostolic Church in Zion Botswana,* Studies on the church in Southern Africa Vol. V, Department of History and Department of Theology and Religious Studies, University of Botswana, 1994.

—. "Healing in the African Independent Churches in the era of HIV/AIDS in Botswana," *Missionalia* Vol. 29:2, 2001, 220-231.

—. "Acceptance and Rejection: The Traditional-Healer Prophet and His Integration of Healing Methods," *BOLESWA Journal of Theology, Religion and Philosophy (BJTRP),* Volume 1:1, 2005, 109-121.

—. "The Church and HIV/AIDS in Africa: an overview and ethical considerations," in Amanze J. N., Nkomazana F. and Kealotswe O. N. (eds) *Christian Ethics and HIV/AIDS in Africa,* Gaborone: Bay Publishing, 2007, 14-27.

Sundkler, G. *Bantu Prophets in South Africa,* London: Oxford University Press, 1961.

Turner, H.W. *African Independent Church, The Life and Faith of the Church of the Lord* (Aladura), Oxford: Clarendon Press, 1967.

West, M. *Bishops and Prophets in a Black City, African Independent Churches in SOWETO,* Cape Town David Philip, 1975.

Interviews

Chidoda, Interview: Gaborone, 23 May 2008
Prophetess Noga, Interview: Gaborone, 30 June 2000
Pudiephatswa, Interview: Gaborone, 25 June 2001

CHAPTER SIX

PENTECOSTAL CHURCHES AND HIV AND AIDS IN BOTSWANA

LOVEMORE TOGARASEI AND FIDELIS NKOMAZANA

Introduction

This chapter discusses the role played by Pentecostal churches in HIV and AIDS response in Botswana. Pentecostal churches make up what one may call a third brand of Christianity, the other two being mainline churches and African Independent Churches (AICs). Mainline churches are those churches that were introduced in Botswana through direct missionary work from the Western world. African Independent Churches, on the other hand, came about as Africans felt dissatisfied with mainline churches and founded their own churches in which they could worship God and still observe certain African cultural practices and beliefs. Pentecostal Churches are known for their teaching on the need to be born-again and the preaching of the gospel of prosperity (that is, a gospel that promotes physical and material well-being). Two types of Pentecostal churches can, however, be identified in Botswana. First, are the classical Pentecostal churches that, like mainline churches, were introduced by missionary Pentecostals from the West, through South Africa. Second, are what one can call charismatic Pentecostal churches, most of which were introduced in Botswana by preachers coming from other African countries like Ghana, Nigeria, Zimbabwe and Malawi. This second type of Pentecostalism which Togarasei (2005) calls 'modern Pentecostalism' is growing very fast in Botswana. This chapter discusses the role played by these Pentecostal churches in HIV and AIDS response. As members of these churches make huge financial contributions to the coffers of the churches (as evident from the high life styles of their leaders), it is important to discuss the role that the churches are playing in a country devastated by HIV and AIDS. How do they view HIV and AIDS, what is their divine message in the light of the suffering caused by the disease? Are they a problem in the fight against HIV and AIDS as Weinrich and Benn (2004:98) say of churches in general? What sex education, if any, do they teach to the youth? What is their attitude towards condom use and how do they address issues of gender? These are some of the questions to be investigated as we pursue to establish the role played by Pentecostal churches in Botswana in HIV and AIDS response.

Data used in this chapter was collected by the two authors in the various research projects they have contacted among Pentecostal churches in Botswana. Two such projects need detailed descriptions since they form the bulk of the data used in this chapter. The first project was the TRS Ditumelo research project whose aim was to assess faith based organizations' (FBOs) capacity to prevent HIV and AIDS in Botswana (Togarasei et. al 2008). Although the project focused on all FBOs in Botswana in seven health districts of the country, this chapter depends on data collected from Pentecostal church responses. The authors isolated Pentecostal responses and analysed the data separately. The other project that forms the bulk of the data for this chapter was carried out by L. Togarasei between 2006 and 2008 and focused specifically on Botswana Pentecostal churches' response to HIV and AIDS. The project is described in detail in the next chapter of this book and will be referred to in this chapter as 'the Togarasei project'.

Pentecostal churches' general views of HIV and AIDS

Pentecostal churches' understanding of HIV and AIDS is mainly influenced by their theology. Believing strongly that God is in control of whatever happens among his people, Pentecostals, like many other Christians, initially believed that HIV and AIDS were diseases for sinners. With this understanding Pentecostal churches were very vocal in accusing those living with HIV of being sinners. Emphasizing morality, they described those living with HIV and AIDS as receiving due punishment from God. The result of this understanding was stigmatization and discrimination of people living with HIV and AIDS (PLWHA). This stigmatization and discrimination was both in word and in deeds. For example in a sermon, one Pentecostal preacher had this to say about PLWHA:

> Imagine your host inviting you for dinner and serving you fish. He eats all the flesh on the fish and then serves you with the skeleton of the fish including its big head! This is typical of someone who turns to God only

when suffering from AIDS. God wants you when you are still health
(Evangelist Peter D. Chiweshe, Video recorded sermon).

Although nearly all churches took this stance (Perry, 2003:11, Chitando
2007:20), Pentecostal churches, with their emphasis on morality and
literalist reading of the Bible were at the forefront of fuelling stigma and
discrimination. Several efforts have since been made on radio, television,
in newspapers and through publication of education programmes by both
governmental and non-governmental organizations to eradicate stigma and
discrimination. These efforts have seen the rate of stigma and discrimination
falling down even among the Pentecostal churches. For example, in a
study of the capacity of FBOs to prevent HIV and AIDS in Botswana,
Togarasei et al (2008) found out that about 3% of Pentecostal respondents
felt that their leaders were weakly committed to discouraging stigma. The
rest (97%) said they believed that their leaders were strongly committed to
discouraging stigma and discrimination. But although statistics paint a
good picture, interacting with the Pentecostals will show that there still
remain traces of stigma and discrimination in these churches. The
experience of these authors while attending Pentecostal church gatherings
is that people living with HIV and AIDS are still stigmatized. Some
pastors' messages concerning HIV and AIDS still condemn people living
with HIV and AIDS for immorality. For example, one of the authors of
this chapter came across a couple living with HIV and AIDS in Gaborone
who left one of the Pentecostal churches because of the stigmatizing and
discriminating messages preached by leaders of the church on people
living with HIV and AIDS. The couple informed him that emphasis was
on being healed and that those who were not healed were not supported
through counseling but were rather accused of being sinners who lacked
faith.   Very few people in these churches have gone public about their
HIV positive status. In interviews, those who have gone public about their
status have mentioned stigmatization as the main obstacle for many people
living with HIV and AIDS not to go public. One of the authors had to
interview a respondent living with HIV and AIDS in private for the
respondent's fear of being known to be living with HIV. Furthermore there
is still the belief that HIV and AIDS is God's way of punishing sinners. In
the Togarasei project to be discussed in detail in the next chapter,
Togarasei found out that 18% (11 out of 60) of the respondents believed
that HIV and AIDS are punishments for immorality, 42 % said their
church leadership did not encourage PLWHA to go public about their HIV
positive status and although 78% said their churches would accept pastors
(ministers) living with HIV and AIDS, 17% said they were not sure if they
could be accepted.

Pentecostal churches in Botswana have also made huge strides in as far as their knowledge of HIV and AIDS is concerned. Even the statistical figures on stigma and discrimination above (3% who felt that their leaders were weakly committed to fighting stigma and discrimination) show that very few Pentecostals are stigmatizing PLWHA. The Togarasei project also showed that 83% of the respondents believed that less than half the number of people in their churches believed that one can get infected with HIV by shaking hands with PLWHA. 78% also believed that less than half the number of members of their congregation believed that a person can get infected with HIV by sharing a meal with a person living with HIV. Nearly all respondents said members of their churches now see HIV and AIDS as any other disease. In interviews, a number of Pentecostals said that God should not be held responsible for HIV and AIDS. They said instead, it is the devil that is responsible for the suffering caused by HIV and AIDS. They said HIV is a spirit send by the devil to torment the people of God.

Pentecostal churches' HIV and AIDS prevention activities

The most common HIV prevention activities promoted by churches are abstinence for those not married and faithfulness in marriage (the so-called A and B methods of HIV prevention). Pentecostal churches are much more rigid when it comes to promoting these two prevention methods when compared to other Christian denominations. The Togarasei project showed that all the 60 respondents to the questionnaire agreed that abstinence and faithfulness in marriage were the prevention activities promoted by their churches. To promote these prevention activities some Pentecostal churches in Botswana teach skills for abstinence and faithfulness. The Evangelical Fellowship of Botswana (EFB), a grouping of Pentecostal and Evangelical churches, for example, runs a project called "True Love Waits" in the district of Ghanzi (www.efbotswana.org). One of the authors interviewed one pastor responsible for running the programme, Pastor Wessels, who said they organize abstinence weekends in partnership with the District Multi-sectoral HIV and AIDS Committee (DMSAC) to provide support to young people who have pledged to abstain until marriage (Interview, April 2007). Through plays, Bible study and talk shows and through art competition, the youths are encouraged to abstain until marriage. The Open Baptist Church (a member of the EFB) in Gaborone also runs the Faith for the Nation Campaign, a programme meant to promote abstinence for those not married. According to Prof. Adedoyin, in a presentation made at the Consultative Meeting on

HIV/AIDS Prevention and Care on 15 September 2008, in 2008 the programme reached out to 9474 youths who made commitments to abstain until marriage. A number of Pentecostal churches also run what they call Marriage Enrichment Seminars which are meant to promote faithfulness in marriage by equipping the married with skills to live faithful lives. According to one elder of the church, the Apostolic Faith Mission for example, conducts regular marriage seminars aimed at promoting faithfulness and abstinence for those not married (Interview, Gaborone, 15 May 2008).

Pentecostal churches in Botswana also promote Prevention of Mother to Child Transmission (PMCT) as a prevention activity. To equip their members with knowledge of HIV and AIDS and thus enable them to prevent infection, 63% of people who completed questionnaires in the Togarasei project agreed that visitors or experts in HIV and AIDS were invited to their churches to discuss HIV prevention with members. Unfortunately some 15% said their churches invited these experts often (nearly every week). The majority (68%) said their churches receive such expert visitors rarely (less than once in a month).

The most widely promoted method of HIV prevention especially in public media in Botswana is the use of condoms. Pentecostal churches are, however, against the promotion of condoms as an HIV prevention method. They believe that this is against the biblical teaching of purity in matters of sex. Only 10% of respondents in a study by Togarasei et al (2008:31) said their church leadership would promote the use of condoms by the unmarried. Along the same line, the Togarasei project also found out that only 13% of the respondents said their churches promoted the government and other organizations' condom distribution programme. Also in a study of four Pentecostal churches in Francistown, T. Mabotho (2008) found out that 20% of her respondents said they would recommend that people should use a condom whenever they are involved in sex before marriage. In interviews Pentecostal church leaders accepted that they knew that there are people who do not abstain and who are not faithful to their partners but they did not want to give mixed messages, "that is, that their congregants should abstain on one hand but carry a condom in their wallet or purse on the other" (Togarasei et al 2008:31). Others, however, said that in counseling sessions they encourage those who cannot abstain to use condoms. Pentecostal churches are, however, strongly opposed to the distribution of condoms among school children. In workshops conducted by the Ditumelo Project Team in 2005 in Selibe-Phikwe and Francistown, Pentecostal churches raised strong objections to the idea of the distribution of condoms to young children especially at primary school (Nkomazana, workshop notes). They saw this as giving these children a license to engage in sexual activities at that tender age. They pointed out that those who were distributing condoms were also undermining and disregarding parental authority by giving children condoms with parents' permission. They also said by giving children condoms, the government was going against the principles of *Botho* (humanness), which is fundamental to the culture and existence of Batswana. They argued that instead of giving them condoms, children must be taught good values and abstinence.

The Pentecostal attitude towards the use of condoms is different when it comes to discordant couples. Nearly all studies in Botswana have shown that Pentecostal churches encourage discordant couples to use condoms. Togarasei et al (2008:30) found out that 54% of Pentecostal respondents said their church leaders promoted the use of condoms by married people. Mabotho (2008:29) found out that 98% of her respondents recommended that married couples with one partner infected should use condoms. Thus the old argument that churches, especially Pentecostal churches, are anti-condom can no longer be sustained. There is a significant number of Pentecostal church members who believe that for the protection of life, condoms should be used by those who cannot abstain or be faithful to their partners. There is also a consensus that discordant couples should use condoms.

Care for the infected and affected

Compared to mainline churches, Botswana Pentecostal churches seem to lag behind in terms of provision of care and support to the infected and affected. It is possible for some Pentecostal churches to go for months without mentioning HIV and AIDS in their sermons. This peripheral treatment of the pandemic is also evident in the churches' programmes and activities. The Togarasei project found out that only 20% of the Pentecostal churches had standing HIV and AIDS committees. The rest did not have such committees. When it comes to care and support as activities, the same study found out that only one out of the five churches ran an orphanage. Although those who did not run orphanages cited lack of funds as the reason for their failure to run such an important programme, it can be concluded that the peripheral treatment of the pandemic is the major cause. The study also established that only one church had a home-based care programe for PLWHA.

But the information above does not, however, mean that Pentecostal churches in Botswana are not providing care and support to PLWHA and those affected. In several interviews conducted by these authors, it was established that the churches provide care and support through their individual members who are taught to be compassionate and loving. Respondents stated that Pentecostal churches, through their members, pray for those in hospitals, clinics and prisons. They make daily or weekly visits to pray and give hope to those who are infected. They also provide food, clothes and avail their various talents and labour to the infected and affected. One church in Palapye stated that their members visit those receiving home based care and minister to them spiritually, emotionally and materially. They discourage stigmatization and discrimination by teaching that HIV and AIDS is like any other disease. In Selibe Phikwe one pastor mentioned that their church members are active members of the villages and wards home based care committees.

Another common way by which Pentecostal churches provide care and support is through counseling. The Apostolic Faith Mission, for example runs counselling sessions every week and according to one elder of the church, there is evidence that many PLWHA attend these sessions and have found them helpful in encouraging them to live positively (Interview, Gaborone, 15/03/2008). The Evangelical Fellowship of Botswana also provides pastoral care to PLWHA. According to Secretary General of the organization, Bishop Owen Isaacs, EFB is also running a research project aimed at finding ways of effectively caring for the infected and affected (Interview, Gaborone, 21/08/2008).   Thus Pentecostal churches are providing care and support to PLWHA and those affected. However, most of these activities are not coordinated by the churches but are left to individual members. As a result the churches' roles are not well documented and therefore cannot be monitored and evaluated together with other national HIV and AIDS responses.

Treatment of PLWHA

The subject of treatment of HIV and AIDS is very controversial when it comes to Pentecostal churches. This is because from the outbreak of the disease, some Pentecostal churches have claimed to be able to cure the disease despite science's declaration that there is no cure. Most Pentecostal churches believe that since "nothing is impossible with God," those with HIV and AIDS can be cured with the virus completely disappearing from the body. There are therefore so many cases of people who claim to have been cured of HIV in Pentecostal churches. Recently the media in Botswana has carried several stories of Pentecostal preachers who urge their members on ARV therapy to get rid of their medicine and trust God for healing. The Sunday Standard of 19 August 2008, for example, reported that police were investigating a case in which a Zimbabwean pastor of the Abundant Life Ministries was deported from Botswana after it was realized that he discouraged members of his church from taking ARV treatment. This is not an isolated case. The Mmegi of 25 May 2007 also reported that police had recovered ARV medication from a site used by one Pentecostal church in Francistown. The police suspected that this was medication thrown away by those who believed only God could cure them. It is, however, not all Pentecostal churches that discourage PLWHA from taking medication. In fact most of the Pentecostal churches encourage those on medication to continue and even take it appropriately as prescribed by medical personnel. The EFB together with the other two Christian organizations in Botswana (the Organization of African Instituted Churches and the Botswana Christian Council), encourage their members on ARVs not to stop taking prescriptions without professional medical advice (http://www.mest.gov.bw/dailynews /news.php). Recently the President of the EFB, Pastor B. Butale had the following to say about ARVs, "Yes there are some members of my church who are on ARV treatment but I have never told them to stop (taking the medication)" (Mmegi Vol 25:30, Wed. 28 February, 2008). He went further to acknowledge that he was aware of some church leaders who discouraged their members from taking ARVs but described this as unfortunate. The Togarasei project also found out that generally Pentecostals do not discourage their members from taking ARVs. Asked if their church leadership encouraged PLWHA to take ARVs, about 80% of the respondents answered in the affirmative. Only 2% said their leadership discouraged members living with HIV and AIDS from taking ARVs.

Pentecostal churches do not only treat HIV and AIDS by encouraging their members to take ARVs. They also believe that through prayer those with HIV and AIDS can be healed with the virus completely disappearing from their bodies. The Togarasei project found out that 83% of the respondents said more than half the members of the churches believed that HIV and AIDS can be healed in the name of God. Respondents said the most common ways by which this healing was practiced in their churches was through the laying on of hands in prayer (97%), through prayers of the leaders of the church (78%) and through use of holy oil (32%). About 60% of the respondents said they had been healed or knew someone who has been healed of HIV and AIDS. Asked what the signs were that one was healed of HIV and AIDS, 83% said those who were healed were declared HIV negative by a medical doctor after the healing process while 33% said all signs of illness had disappeared. In interviews the respondents stated that those healed of HIV and AIDS had initially been medically declared to be infected.

Despite faith healing and encouraging PLWHA to take ARVs, Pentecostals in Botswana also mention that they treat the infected by providing and encouraging the infected to eat healthy foods. The EFB runs a vegetable project in Masunga which provides healthy food to those receiving home based care in the village (Mmegi, Vol 25:30, Wed. 28 February, 2008). Pentecostal churches together with other Christian organizations also provide pastoral care and counseling to give hope to the infected by encouraging them to put their faith in God and to accept their condition and live positively. They also encourage the infected to take physical exercises in order to keep healthy.

Pentecostal hindrances and weaknesses to effective HIV and AIDS response

Our discussion of Pentecostal response above shows that Pentecostal churches in Botswana are in some ways involved in HIV and AIDS national response. They are involved in prevention, in care and support of the infected and affected and in the treatment of the infected. However, when one compares the large membership of these churches and the commitment generally expressed by Pentecostals towards Christian life, one can easily notice a mismatch when it comes to commitment to HIV and AIDS response. There are a number of possible reasons that cause this lack of serious commitment. Let us consider some of these reasons.

Spiritualization of the problem

Some Pentecostal churches in Botswana spiritualise the HIV and AIDS pandemic by referring to it as a demon or as spiritual possession. Such understandings of the pandemic are often made in sermons. At one Pentecostal church service in Gaborone, one pastor had this to say, "It is good for us as a church to welcome people infected by HIV. However, the God I worship is not a God of the ill. The demon called HIV should therefore be cast out in the name of Jesus." This attitude leads not only to stigmatization of HIV and AIDS but also to the church putting too much effort in dealing with the pandemic spiritually than physically. It probably explains why a number of Pentecostal churches, particularly the charismatic ones, do not have structures to deal with the social problems caused by HIV and AIDS. Emphasis is put on healing without looking at other forms of response like establishment of orphanages and provision of home based care programmes. HIV and AIDS is also a result of many other social issues like, the abuse of women and children, poverty, unequal access to resources, discriminatory workplace practices and so. By spiritualizing the HIV and AIDS problems, Pentecostal churches lose sight of the need to address these social problems.

Claims that HIV and AIDS can be cured

Related to the spiritualization of HIV and AIDS as a cause of Pentecostal lack of serious commitment to HIV and AIDS response is the belief that in the name of God, HIV can be cured. That Pentecostals believe that HIV and AIDS can be cured is testified by several studies. We have seen above that 80% of respondents in the Togarasei project believed that HIV and AIDS can be cured. In his preliminary study of Pentecostal churches and HIV/AIDS in Nigeria, J. Smith (2006) attended healing ceremonies in which infected members of the church were 'healed' with some churches having teams of 'prayer warriors' who pray all day for the cure of their fellow church members (www.watsoninstitute.org/news, accessed 29/01/09). Indeed there are several cases of people who have claimed that they have been cured of HIV and AIDS by Pentecostal healers. Without questioning Pentecostal claims to cure HIV and AIDS, this attitude again draws the churches' attention to physical healing leaving them not committed to other forms of HIV and AIDS response. Instead of providing care and support to PLWHA, Pentecostal churches would then put more emphasis on healing, which more often than note, does not take place. Emphasis on healing also promotes stigmatization as those who are not healed are often accused of lacking faith.

Lack of resources

Botswana Pentecostal churches also lack resources to effectively respond to HIV and AIDS. This is not because members cannot afford to raise resources for responding to HIV and AIDS, but because the leadership is not seriously committed to HIV and AIDS response. The Togarasei project found out that most modern Pentecostal churches in Botswana did not have fund raising projects earmarked to raise financial and other resources for HIV and AIDS response. Only 5% of the respondents said their churches had submitted a funding proposal for HIV activities to a trust, foundation or government in the two years preceding the conducting of this research. The churches also did not have posters or pamphlets displayed in their buildings to conscientize members about HIV and

AIDS. Only 30% of the respondents said some members of their churches had received training on behalf of the church on any HIV related programmes in the one year preceding the conducting of this research project. Such statistics surely shows that Pentecostal churches in Botswana have not yet put HIV and AIDS at the centre of their activities despite the havoc it has caused in the Botswana society.

Fundamentalism

Pentecostals can be described as fundamentalist in their approach to faith. We do not, however, use the term fundamentalism in a pejorative way like R. Dawkins (2006: cited in wikpedia.rog/wiki/Fundamentalism, accessed 2/02/09) who uses it to characterise religious advocates as clinging to a stubborn, entrenched position that defies reasoned argument or contradictory evidence. Rather by fundamentalism here we mean a conservative Christian position with a strong emphasis on conservative values, the inerrancy of the Bible and a literal approach to its interpretation (Tate 2006:146). Pentecostals uphold conservative moral teachings of abstinence and faithfulness in marriage. As a result, they do not want to entertain any ideas of condom use for those not married. This position, however, does not cater for those who may fail to observe the conservative morality. It is indeed very true that there are many members of Pentecostal churches that fail to live by the churches' moral teachings. In Botswana this is evidenced by the fact that many people have children out of wedlock. Some Pentecostal churches even have 'Single Mothers Fellowship Groups,' an acceptance by the churches that there are people who have children out of wedlock. Of course this is not to deny that some single mothers are in that condition because of divorce or they have been widowed. However, the underlying factor is that churches, including Pentecostals are not full of saints but also abound with those who fail to live by the moral codes. For us, the churches must adopt a theology which is life affirming and which leaves sinners with a second chance to repent while they are still not infected. Pentecostals therefore need to reevaluate their attitude towards condom use for those who are not married and who fail to live by the churches' strict moral code.

Marginal involvement of women in decision making structures

Although the rise of Pentecostalism in the early 20th century saw the greater involvement of women in church affairs (Burgess, *Encyclopedia of Pentecostal and Charismatic Christianity,* 460), this was not to remain so.

In Botswana very few Pentecostal churches are led by women. Togarasei (2006:127) explains the position of women in these churches, "Although the churches have appointed women as a pastors, their voices are not as strong as those of the male pastors. In most cases women play the roles of ushers, flower arrangers and Sunday school teachers." Considering that women are affected by HIV and AIDS more than men (Dube 2003), this marginal involvement of women in decision making positions, probably explains the marginalization of HIV and AIDS in Pentecostal churches activities.

Conclusion and way forward

In this chapter we have discussed Pentecostal churches response to HIV and AIDS in Botswana. Focusing mainly on modern/charismatic Pentecostal churches, it has been noted that the churches are playing some roles in HIV prevention, care and support and treatment of those infected and affected. The chapter has also shown that there are specific hindrances to effective Pentecostal response. Some of the hindrances identified are spiritualisation of the problem, claims to be able to cure the disease, fundamentalism, lack of resources and gender inequity in decision making positions. As a way forward, we therefore suggest that Pentecostal churches need to seriously commit themselves to HIV and AIDS response as the pandemic is not only affecting potential members of the churches but also those who are already members of these churches. The churches should accept the reality of the problem and instead of spiritualizing the problem, they should "come down to earth" and address HIV and AIDS in the same way they address the need for material prosperity. This is because when it comes to material possessions in the here and now, Pentecostals are at the forefront of promoting this doctrine. They teach that believers will not only receive rewards from God in heaven, but are also blessed materially here on earth through money, cars, houses and other forms of wealth. Modern Pentecostals are therefore known for upholding an ethic of hard work in order to become wealthy and prove the gospel of prosperity correct. It is unfortunate that when it comes to responding to HIV and AIDS, the same effort is not promoted to provide for the physical well-being of the infected and affected.

Bibliography

Adedoyin, A. Faith the Nation, powerpoint presentation notes, 15 September, 2008.

Burgess, S.M. (ed.). *Encyclopedia of Pentecostal and Charismatic Christianity,* New York: Routledge, 2006.

Chitando, E. *Living With Hope: African Churches and HIV/AIDS Vol. 1,* Geneva: WCC Publications, 2007.

Dube, M. W. Culture, Gender and HIV/AIDS: Understanding and Acting on the Issues, in Dube, M. W. (ed.) *HIV/AIDS and the Curriculum: Methods of Integrating HIV/AIDS in Theological Programmes,* Geneva: WCC Publications, 2003, 85-100.

Mabotho, T. *The Position of Pentecostal Churches on the use of condoms in the HIV and AIDS Era,* Unpublished B.A. dissertation, Department of Theology and Religious Studies, University of Botswana, 2008.

Mmegi Vol 25:30, Wed. 28 February, 2008

Mmegi, Vol. 24:167, 25 May 2007.

Perry, S. *Responses of the Faith-Based Organizations to HIV/AIDS in Sub-Saharan Africa,* Geneva: World Council of Churches, 2003.

Tate, W. R. *Interpreting the Bible: A Handbook of Methods and Terms,* Peabody: Hendrikson Publishers, 2006.

Togarasei, L."Modern Pentecostalism as an Urban Phenomenon: the case of the Family of God Church in Zimbabwe," *Exchange: Journal of Missiological and Ecumenical Studies,* Vol.34:4, 2005, 349-375.

Togarasei, L. *et al, An Assessment of the Capacity of Faith-based organizations for HIV prevention in Botswana,* Gaborone: Associated Printers, 2008.

Weinreich, S. and Benn, C. *AIDS: Meeting the Challenge,* Geneva: WCC Publications, 2004.

Other sources

Apostolic Faith Mission Elder, Interview: Gaborone, 15/03/2008

Bishop Owen Isaacs, Interview: Gaborone, 21/08/2008

Pastor Wessels, Interview: Ghanzi, April 2007

Chiweshe, P. D. (2002), Kutenda Chinyi? Video recorded sermon

www.efbotswana.org, accessed 2/02/09

http://www.mest.gov.bw/dailynews/news.php, accessed 28/03/09

www.watsoninstitute.org/news, accessed 29/01/09

wikpedia.rog/wiki/Fundamentalism, accessed 2/02/09

CHAPTER SEVEN

THE USE OF THE BIBLE IN HIV AND AIDS CONTEXTS: CASE STUDY OF SOME PENTECOSTAL CHURCHES IN BOTSWANA

LOVEMORE TOGARASEI

Introduction

Between October 2006 and February 2008 the Ditumelo Research Team of the Department of Theology and Religious Studies, University of Botswana undertook an assessment of the capacity of faith-based organizations (FBOs) to prevent HIV in Botswana (Togarasei, et al 2008). One of the methods we used to gather data was district participatory workshops. The workshops began with various activities meant to identify what FBOs considered to be major factors contributing to the spread of HIV in their district, what they were doing as faith communities and what their obstacles were. They were then followed by discussions in which the research team wanted to get clarifications on certain responses that came out from the participatory activities. It is in these discussions that I, as a biblical scholar, noted the continued surfacing of the Bible and what it teaches. Although we were not interested in discussions on what the role of the Bible is in responses to HIV since we were assessing all faiths not Christianity alone, on account of their large numbers, Christians often brought up the Bible and how it shapes their responses to HIV and AIDS. I realized that the most vocal participants on this subject were from Pentecostal churches. Often they would declare, "But the Bible says….." I had just been granted a research grant by the Office of Research and Development of the University of Botswana to find out the role of Pentecostal churches in HIV response in Botswana. I therefore took advantage of this to bring in the issue of the role of the Bible in HIV and

AIDS contexts. The article is based on this research that I undertook between August 2007 and August 2008 among Pentecostal churches. This is the project we have referred to as the 'Togarasei project' in the preceding chapter. This chapter therefore seeks to analyse the use of the Bible by Pentecostal churches in Botswana in contexts of HIV and AIDS. How has the Bible shaped the responses of these Christian communities to HIV and AIDS?, is the question at the centre of the article. It is also the intention of this chapter to go further and look at how the Bible can continue to be used in contexts of HIV and AIDS. But before delving into the central question of the use of the Bible in HIV and AIDS contexts, there is need to give a brief background of the place of the Bible in Africa. It is after appreciating the place of the Bible generally in Africa that one can then understand its use among Pentecostal churches in HIV and AIDS contexts in Botswana. The chapter is therefore divided into four sections. The first section, as already stated, looks at the general use and place of the Bible in Africa. The second section discusses the methodology of my study of the use of the Bible among Pentecostal churches in Botswana. The third section presents the results of this study. The fourth section discusses the results before a conclusion of the chapter is given.

The Bible in Africa

Let me begin by specifying that by Africa here I mean sub-Saharan/Tropical Africa and particularly southern Africa. The use of the Bible in this region dates back to almost two centuries ago through Coptic and Ethiopian communities (Holter 2000:9). From that period to this day, the Bible has deeply influenced the people of Africa. It has become a book that Africans hold very dearly to their hearts. As Mbiti (2005:234-248) says, Bible reading in Africa has become a mass movement. S. Nadar (2007) refers to Desmond Tutu's joke that even if colonizers had stolen all African land and left Africans with the Bible, Africans would be better off. Although just a joke, and one which many Africans would dispute, it sheds much light on the place of the Bible in Africa. Indeed Bible reading is a mass movement in Africa. The Bible, as Mbiti (2005:234-248) sub-titles his article, has found a place in "African homes, schools and churches." What Beasley *et al* (1991:26-28) say about the general approaches to Bible study is very true of the way the Bible is used in Africa. The most common approach is what they call the devotional/religious approach. This is the reading of the Bible to enrich personal faith. Here reading can be done individually, by a family, in small Bible study groups and also at church gatherings. The Bible is therefore the only book that one is likely to find in every home, be it a Christian or non-Christian home. Sermons which do not refer to the Bible are more likely to be criticized by listeners. In the devotional approach, the Bible is believed to be the Word of God containing guidelines on personal and spiritual growth. For many who approach the Bible from this perspective, the Bible has readymade answers to human problems. They therefore approach it, "with an attitude of reverence and prayer, asking that God's Spirit lead them in their study" (Beasley *et al* 1991:26). Nadar (2007) goes further explaining the centrality of the Bible among Africans. She says:

> ....the Bible is also a book of comfort and resources for daily living for African Christians. People look to it for daily inspiration. It is not uncommon for people to read a verse or a chapter each day for encouragement and comfort. The Bible is also used as a guide for daily living and spiritual direction. In other words, when Christians are faced with moral dilemmas they are likely to reach for the Bible to see what it has to say about the challenge they are facing.

Nadar also notes the magical use of the Bible in Africa. She refers to how, according to Mercy Amba Oduyoye, the Bible is put in babies' cots in West Africa to ward off evil spirits. The magical use of the Bible is also practiced mainly by African Independent Churches' (AICs) prophets when it is placed upon the ill as a healing method. Among these churches, M. Dube (2000:67-80; 2006:193-207) has also discovered the divinatory use of the Bible. The method is influenced by the African practice of throwing bones or other divining objects to diagnose human problems and to find answers to these problems. Dube noted that in the same way bones or other such divining objects were used by traditional healers, Christians in AICs used biblical texts. Instead of throwing bones, AICs prophets would hand the Bible to the patient, ask her to open whatever text and hand it back to the prophet. Through interpretation of the opened text the prophet then divines the problems of the patient and offers the remedy (Togarasei 2008:55-74).

Another approach to the use of the Bible discussed by Beasley *et al* (1991) is the scholarly/critical approach. This description is a bit misleading as it assumes that other methods like magical and confessional uses are not critical. Although it may be true from a Western perspective of biblical interpretation, African biblical scholars like J. S. Ukpong (2002:9-40) and M. W. Dube (2006:193-208) find even the devotional approach to be a critical reading of the Bible. This so-called critical approach emphasizes the meaning of the biblical texts in their original settings and is therefore often used in schools, seminaries and universities. It is not a very popular approach in Africa as many of those who use the Bible hear it speaking to their lives and therefore are not interested in its original meaning.

Since this chapter looks at Pentecostal churches' use of the Bible in contexts of HIV and AIDS, it focuses mainly on the devotional use of the Bible. It therefore looks at the use of the Bible as a motivation for personal, group and even national well-being.

The use of the Bible for HIV response by Botswana Pentecostal churches

Having seen how the Bible is used in Africa, let us then turn to consider how Botswana Pentecostal churches have used the Bible in the HIV and AIDS context. The data for this discussion was collected through fieldwork. Therefore below, I discuss first, the background to the project and the methodology employed. This will then be followed by the presentation of the results. I will end with a discussion of the results before the conclusion to the chapter is given.

Background and Methodology of the study

Data used in this article was collected between August 2007 and August 2008 as part of a project on modern Pentecostal churches and HIV and AIDS in Botswana. Modern Pentecostal churches, also referred to just as 'new' Pentecostalism (Gifford 1998, Anderson 2004), charismatic Pentecostalism (Dijk 2004), Charismatic Ministries (Asamoah-Gyadu 2005), or just new or neo-Pentecostal churches (Dada 2004) have taken the Botswana religious landscape by storm. Statistics on Christian identities in Botswana are scarce. Amanze (1994) and Melton (2002), who have done some statistics on religions in Botswana, lump all Christians together (Amanze) or only distinguish Roman Catholic, Protestants and African Independent Churches (Melton). Be that as it may, Togarasei et al (2008) put the Pentecostal churches population at 28% of 572 churches they mapped in 7 health districts of the country. This percentage shows a substantial growth in Pentecostalism considering that for a long time Main line churches and African Independent Churches dominated the Botswana Christian landscape (see Haron 2007:322-339). Pentecostal churches are generally attracting the rich and affluent in Botswana or those who feel they are on a journey to success in life. They are known for preaching a 'healthy and wealthy' gospel (i.e. a gospel that promotes physical well-being and material prosperity) and so this project sought to find out the roles of these churches in HIV and AIDS national response. The project was funded by the Office of Research and Development of the University of Botswana and it sought to:

- find out the role played by modern Pentecostal churches in the fight against HIV and AIDS in Botswana.
- find out, through an analysis of their role, the theology that informs the churches' attitude to HIV and AIDS.
- suggest ways by which the churches can continue to be partners in the fight against the HIV and AIDS pandemic.

There are many modern Pentecostal churches in Botswana hence purposive sampling was used to select churches for study. Criteria were set for this purposive sampling. First, was the size of the church and its geographical spread. Churches with large memberships (those with at least one hundred members and are found in more than five villages or cities in Botswana) were selected. Second, to reflect the rural-urban divide in Botswana, churches with membership both in urban and rural areas were selected. Since the project sought to study Pentecostal view of and contribution to the fight against HIV and AIDS, it is only from these large churches that generalizations could justly be made. On the basis of the set criteria the following churches were selected for the study: Bible Life Ministries, Family of God Church, Forward in Faith, Winners' Chapel and End Time Ministries. The towns and villages in which the study was conducted are: Gaborone, Francistown, Tonota, Palapye-Serowe, Selibe-Phikwe, Ramotswa, Molepolole and Chadibe. Because the intention of the study was to find out the role played by these churches in the fight against HIV and AIDS, data was collected from the church leadership and church members, those affected and infected by HIV.

Four different instruments were used to gather data. To get data from church leaders, interviews were conducted using a designed interview guide. The same method (but with different interview guides) was also used to gather data from those infected and affected by HIV and AIDS. In each church one leader, one person living with HIV and one person affected by HIV or AIDS were interviewed from each town or village. All these respondents were randomly selected with the assistance of the congregations pastors who knew those infected or affected. Questionnaires were used to gather data from the general membership of the churches. Again these were randomly selected with the assistance of the respective pastors of the congregations. All questionnaires were interviewer administered.

A total of 60 respondents (29 Female and 31 Male) completed the questionnaire. Their ages ranged from 20 to 65 years with 34 (about 56%) being in the 20-30 years age range. Most of them (34= 56%) had been members of their respective churches for over two years. It is section 6 of the questionnaire which is of relevance in this chapter. Below is that section of the questionnaire with the questions as they were asked:

Section 6: Biblical interpretation in the age of HIV and AIDS

No.	Questions	Responses	Code
700	The solution to the problem of HIV and AIDS lies in the Bible: Would members of your church agree?	1. Yes 2. No 3. Do not know	
701	If Yes, state two ways in which the Bible can provide a solution to the problem of HIV and AIDS.		
702	If No, which of the following responses would you consider to be nearest to your church's position?	1. The Bible does not mention the word HIV/AIDS 2. The Bible promotes stigma	
703	Which Biblical passages would you say are used in your church to promote the church's HIV prevention activities? (**Briefly explain how they are used**)		
704	Which Biblical passages would you say are used in your church to promote the church's healing activities? (**Briefly explain how they are used**)		
705	Which Biblical passages would you say are used in your church to promote the church's care activities? (**Briefly explain how they are used**)		
706	State any other ways the Bible is used to address HIV and AIDS in your church		

Whereas it was easier to find respondents for the questionnaires, the same was not true for the interviews. Pastors themselves were difficult to find as some of them did not turn up for interviews as scheduled and others would cancel appointments several times. People living with HIV and AIDS (PLWHA) and those infected were reluctant to be interviewed. All in all only 25 of the envisaged 40 interviewees were finally interviewed. Of these, 13 (13 male and 0 female) were pastors, 5 (2 male and 3 female) were PLWHA while the remaining 7 (1 male and 6 female) were people affected by HIV and AIDS. The majority of the interviewees (64%) was aged between 31 and 40 years and had been members of their respective churches for between 2 and 20 years. The PLWH and those affected held different positions in their churches, from general membership to elders. There were no specific questions on the Bible and HIV and AIDS on the infected and affected people interview guides. Thus this chapter makes use of data only from the sections of the pastors' interview guide that dealt with use of the Bible in contexts of HIV and AIDS. Below are those sections in bold:

2.1 What HIV and AIDS Prevention methods does your church promote for:
a) Youth?
b) Women?
c) Men?
d) All members in general
2.2 Which biblical or other teachings influence the methods the church promotes? Explain.

3.1 What Care programmes for the infected and affected people does your church promote?
3.2 Which biblical or other teachings influence the church's involvement in these programmes? Explain

Study Results

The use of the Bible for HIV prevention

Results, both from the questionnaires and from interviews with pastors, show that modern Pentecostal churches in Botswana use the Bible to promote two prevention methods: abstinence for those not married and faithfulness to one partner for those who are married. The texts mentioned in the interviews can therefore be divided into these two prevention methods. The commonly cited text for promotion of abstinence was 2 Timothy 2:22, "So shun youthful passions and aim at righteousness, ..." Respondents emphasized the fact that all those who are not married should not be involved in sexual activities noting that if all in society would give heed to this teaching, there would be little to no transmission of HIV. Also cited to promote abstinence was 1 Corinthians 7:8, "To the unmarried and the widows I say that it is well for them to remain single as I do." As one pastor said in interpretation of the passage, "Paul did not engage in sex, therefore by using his example, he was teaching single Christians not to engage in sex." Other texts used to promote abstinence among the unmarried are all those texts that teach against fornication and adultery: Exodus 20:14, Leviticus 20:20, Deuteronomy 5:18, Matthew 5:27-28, Romans 7:7 (You shall not commit adultery), Galatians 5:19 (Now the works of the flesh are plain: fornication, impurity, ...).

As a prevention measure, Christians are encouraged to get married. Again the Bible is the basis for this teaching. A number of texts were cited by the respondents as the basis for their teaching on marriage. Genesis 2:18 was the commonly cited passage, "Then the Lord God said, "It is not good that the man should be alone, I will make him a helper fit for him." This was often combined together with 1 Corinthians 7:9, "But if they cannot exercise self-control, they should marry." One questionnaire respondent explained these passages further saying that God provides an alternative to those who cannot abstain. This alternative, the respondent said, was marriage. Other texts cited to support marriage are 1 Thessalonians 4:4 (...that each of you know how to take a wife for himself in holiness and honour not in the passion of lust) and 1 Corinthians 7:2 (But because of the temptation to immorality, each man should have his own wife, and each woman her own husband).

Respondents underlined that for marriage to be an effective HIV prevention measure there should be faithfulness between the married. Several biblical texts were cited to support faithfulness. The most common text was 1 Corinthians 7:2-3, "But because of the temptation to immorality, each man should have his own wife and each woman her own husband. The husband should give to his wife her conjugal rights, and likewise the wife to her own husband." Texts against adultery (already mentioned above) were used also to promote faithfulness. Proverbs 6: 24-27 which teaches against prostitution and 1 Corinthians 7:10-11, which teaches against divorce were also cited. One respondent explained that divorce also contributes to the spread of HIV and so if people would give heed to the biblical teaching against divorce, the spread of HIV would be curtailed.

Modern Pentecostal churches also use the Bible to address factors that they perceive to contribute to unfaithfulness among married couples. One such factor mentioned mainly by male respondents and by elderly women was the unsubmissiveness of wives to their husbands. The other factor mentioned was husbands' lack of love towards their wives. The understanding among those who cited these factors was that if a man is not respected by his wife, he is likely to seek extra-marital relationships. Though this sounds very patriarchal and androcentric, it has been confirmed by studies on masculinity elsewhere. Baker and Ricardo (2005) in a study of young men and construction of masculinity in Sub-Saharan Africa, for example, noted that men who felt that their wives did not respect them because they were not employed, tended to have extra-marital relationships. To address wives who are not submissive to their husbands, biblical passages like Ephesians 5:22 and 1 Peter 3 are therefore read, "Wives be submissive to your husbands as to the Lord." They also believe that some women seek extra-marital relationships (thus putting themselves and their partners at risk of HIV) because their husbands do not show them love. Our respondents said to address this, texts like Colossians 3:19 are used, "Husbands, love your wives, and do not be harsh with them."

Other texts are also used to promote abstinence and faithfulness. 1 Corinthians 3:16 and 6:15 which talk of the bodies of Christians as the temple of God were highlighted. One respondent explained. "According to these scriptures, the bodies of Christians are members of Christ, his holy temple. This means the bodies must be kept holy. Keeping one's body holy will therefore protect one from HIV and AIDS." Threats are also used to promote abstinence and faithfulness. One respondent mentioned how they use the story of David's sin with Bathsheba (2 Samuel 12) to show that God punishes sinners. According to the story, God was angry when David committed adultery and murder at the same time. He later had to punish him together with his family. From this story, explained the respondent, Christians must learn that God can punish them for their sins and HIV can be one such punishment for sin. Another respondent even described sexual immorality as leading not only to risks of HIV but also to demonic possession. Using the Pauline teaching that when you commit adultery you become one flesh with the person you are committing it with, the respondent said, "You become one person with that person and so you also expose yourself to demon possession." Reference to HIV and AIDS as God's punishment was also mentioned by some respondents using texts like Jeremiah 30:12-13 (For thus says the Lord: Your heart is incurable and your wound is grievous. There is none to uphold your cause, no medicine for your wound, no healing for you) and Romans 6:23 (For the wages of sin is death, but the free gift of God is eternal life in Christ Jesus our Lord).

The use of the Bible for Care and support

Care and support of the weak and marginalized has been the work of churches for the greater part of Christianity's history. In a number of countries in Africa, churches run health institutions for care and treatment. In Zimbabwe, for example, churches run about 68% of the country's health services (Weinreich and Benn 2004:101). Although not to the same extent as in Zimbabwe, in Botswana churches from the beginning of their missionary work ran health institutions (Mgadla 2007:115-154). This study on Pentecostal churches and HIV and AIDS also found out that these churches emphasise care and support of the infected and affected. Although none of the studied churches were running health institutions like medical clinics or hospitals, treatment, care and support of the infected is central to the missions of the churches. The Bible is read to underscore this need to care and support.

Often used to justify the churches' care and support work was the figure of Jesus. Respondents noted that Jesus did not only care for those who were ill, he especially taught his followers to have a caring attitude. Nearly all respondents cited Jesus' eschatological teaching in Matthew 25:31-46. For these respondents, the passage provides the most compelling criterion upon which the last judgment will be carried out. This criterion is the care and support of the hungry, the thirst, the homeless, the naked, the sick and the imprisoned, in short, those in need. It teaches that in providing care and support to the marginalized and the weak, who in the context of the respondents included the HIV and AIDS infected and affected, they will be doing this to Jesus. In support of Jesus' caring attitude and his teaching that his followers should also be caring and supporting, the parable of the Good Samaritan (Luke 10: 25-37) was also referred to by respondents. As one respondent explained, "The parable teaches Christians to be Good Samaritans wherever they are. They should take care of the ill, whether they have been attacked by thieves or are receiving home based care." Another respondent said, their care activities include providing even financial resources to meet the needs of those infected in their communities. She said in her church, Mark 10:45 which says Jesus came to serve rather than to be served, encourages them to serve the infected and affected, whether church members or non-members, in their neighbourhood.

The biblical teachings on love (Luke 10:27, John 13:34-35, 15:12, Romans 12:9-12) were also cited to support the churches' care and support work. Respondents explained that since God is love and calls upon all to love, Christians are compelled to care and support those infected and affected by HIV and AIDS. One respondent defined love as, "The ability to support those who are in need." Respondents also mentioned that the Bible teaches them not only to love in word, but indeed in their deeds. The spirit of sharing as done by the early church in Jerusalem (Acts 4:32-37) was given as an example to be followed in support of those infected and affected by HIV and AIDS. Acts 9:36-42 which gives an account of Tabitha's works of charity was also cited by many respondents as another basis for the need for Christian care and support of the marginalized. This text was cited together with other passages that encourage works of charity among the poor. One pastor explained that Christians are encouraged to care for and support those infected and affected by HIV and AIDS as in doing that they will be serving God who in turn will reward them. He cited Luke 6:38 as one of those texts used to encourage generous services to the needy, "Give and it will be given to you, good measure, pressed down, shaken together, running over, will be put into your lap. For the measure you give will be the measure you get back." Many other biblical texts were also cited by respondents as texts used to encourage Christians to have compassion towards the HIV and AIDS infected and affected: Matthew 6:1-3 (give without sounding a trumpet and God will reward you), Galatians 6:2 (bear each other's burden), Ephesians 4:4 (Christians are one body of Christ and so they should care for each other).

Christians also use the Bible to counsel the infected and affected. Several biblical texts used for counseling as Christian support were cited. Top on the list of these texts was, however, the story of Job. Biblical scholars have noted two themes in the book of Job: the traditional interpretation of the need to remain faithful under suffering based on the prose section of the book and the modern interpretation of theodicy based on the poetic section (Anderson 1993:8-10). All the respondents said they read the book of Job to highlight the need to remain faithful under suffering. Just as Job lost everything and suffered poor health but remained faithful to God, those infected by HIV are also encouraged to remain faithful to God even in poor health. Respondents also said the infected are encouraged to put faith in God for their healing as the following section shows.

The use of the Bible for Healing

It is in their claim to have powers to heal HIV and AIDS that Pentecostal churches have been criticized by medical scientists. The Ugandan Monitor recently carried an article entitled *Spiritual Healing Threatening Adherence to Antiretrovirals* (www.kaisernetwork.org: accessed 17/10/08). This is because Pentecostals believe that HIV and AIDS can be healed in the name of Jesus. Compared to the other two areas of HIV and AIDS responses discussed above, the respondents gave a lot of scriptural references as evidence to support the healing of HIV and AIDS. We were clear to first find out the respondents' understanding of healing and for almost all of them, HIV and AIDS healing meant the absence of the virus from the body of a previously infected person.

Most of the respondents started by quoting Luke 1:37, "For with God nothing will be impossible." Of the 13 pastors interviewed, 10 (about 77%) cited this scripture as the starting point for the belief that with faith in God the HIV and AIDS infected can be healed. References were also made to the healing of people with leprosy in the Bible (2 Kings 5:1ff, Luke 5:12-16). Respondents explained that just as God healed people with leprosy which was also considered to be incurable then, he still has the power to heal those with HIV and AIDS. After all they quoted, 'God said, "I am the Lord, your healer"' (Exodus 15:26). Another widely cited text was Psalms 103:3 (Bless the Lord, ..., who heals all your diseases). The word 'all' was emphasized by the respondents who referred to this scripture. One respondent to the questionnaire explained, "This scripture means God heals all diseases since *all* include HIV and AIDS." Similarly Isaiah 53:5 (...with his stripes we are healed...) was also cited as evidence that God heals HIV and AIDS. Respondents were categorical that the Bible does not categorise diseases or state that there are certain diseases that are beyond the power of God. They said since HIV and AIDS are illnesses like tuberculosis, cancer or leprosy, God has the power to heal them. One respondent had this to say, "HIV/AIDS can be healed because it is a disease like any other disease. In this regard, it can be healed. There is no weapon planned against us that can prosper. The word of God is sharper than any two-edged sword and it is alive up to today." Hebrews

13:8 (Jesus Christ is the same yesterday, today and forever) was used to argue that if Jesus healed all diseases and that he does not change, it means he is able to heal HIV and AIDS as well. Since he has given power to his followers to heal (Mark 16:17-And these signs will accompany those who believe…..they will lay their hands on the sick and they will recover), respondents were unanimous that today's church has the power to heal HIV and AIDS.

The Bible was also used to prescribe healing methods. Mark 14:17 and Acts 9:17-19 were cited as prescribing the laying on of hands in prayer as a healing method. James 5:14 was cited as the scriptural reference for the use of oil for healing.

Discussion

"There is no mention of HIV/AIDS in the Hebrew Bible," writes J. Stiebert (2003:30). The same is true of the New Testament. The whole Bible does not mention HIV and AIDS as it did not exist when the biblical books were written (Happonen 2005:128). However, as we have seen above, Pentecostal churches in Botswana find the Bible very useful in responding to HIV and AIDS. They use the Bible to understand the suffering and loss caused by HIV and AIDS, to prevent contraction of the virus, to care for those infected and affected and to heal those infected and affected. As one respondent said, "The Bible is the manual for our lives in everything even on HIV and AIDS." What is clear therefore is that although the Bible does not mention HIV and AIDS, because of its place and authority in Pentecostal churches, Christians make what Happonen (2005:128) calls "extended application" between genuinely comparable situations we find in biblical times and our circumstances today. Pentecostal churches consider the Bible to be the inspired word of God. Bible reading and applications to situations in life is therefore central to members of these churches. As one Pentecostal theologian writes, "For Pentecostals, the thought and praxis of the tradition has been and continues to be informed directly by the biblical texts themselves" (Thomas 1998:310). Because of this tradition, questions about HIV and AIDS are therefore answered from the perspective of the Bible. This results in what we experienced in the district workshops I mentioned above, "But the Bible says….." Following this method of using the Bible, one can easily understand churches, and particularly Pentecostal churches' initial reactions to the outbreak of HIV and AIDS. Let us briefly revisit this initial understanding to see the role that the Bible played in responding to HIV and AIDS.

As they often do, when HIV and AIDS broke out, churches sought a biblical answer to the problem. This they found mainly in the biblical, specifically Deuteronomic, doctrine that teaches that God rewards the righteous and punishes sinners (Deuteronomy 7:12-15). As many scholars (for example, Togarasei 2002:254-271, Kgalemang 2004:141-168, Munyika 2005:74-117, Chitando 2007:21) have lamented, this reading of the Bible perpetuated stigmatization and discrimination. PLWHA were seen as sinners receiving their due punishment for their sins. Informed by their reading of the Bible, churches, especially Pentecostal churches also became associated with rigid sexual morality and the rejection of prevention measures like use of condoms, sexual education for youth and rigid gender roles (Weinreich and Benn 2004:98). In fact all the accusations that were leveled against churches in their response to HIV and AIDS (e.g. being a "sleeping giant", promoting stigma and discrimination based on fear and prejudice, pronouncing harsh moral judgments on those infected, obstructing the efforts of the secular world in the area of prevention and reducing the issues of AIDS to simplistic moral pronouncements (Perry 2003:3)) were to a large extent a result of their reading of the Bible.

This chapter shows that Pentecostals have not read the Bible only to stigmatise the infected. In fact, it is the understanding in these churches that this reading (that HIV activists thought promoted stigma) is meant to prevent HIV and AIDS. As we noted in the presentation of results above, Pentecostal churches believe the threat of God's punishment for adultery/fornication should stop people from engaging in HIV risk behaviours. For them, the role of the church is to encourage people to live by the standards of God. It is in leading godly lives that people can prevent themselves from contracting the virus. It is the Pentecostals' use of the Bible that explains their attitude to condom use as a method of HIV prevention. Earlier studies of Pentecostal churches in Botswana (Mabotho 2008, Togarasei et al 2008) show that less than 50% of Pentecostal churches membership believe that condoms can be used outside marriage. Influenced by their reading of the Bible which promotes abstinence for the unmarried and faithfulness for the married, many Pentecostals are against talk of condom use for the unmarried.

It is therefore my conviction that responses to HIV and AIDS by governments and non-governmental organizations (NGOs) should take seriously the influence that the Bible has among Christians, particularly those from the Pentecostal churches. As noted above, Pentecostal churches take seriously the authority of the Bible. They believe that God was revealed to humanity through Scripture. They consider the Bible to be the inspired Word of God (2 Timothy 3:16), inerrant and authoritative (Decker 2006:25-61). Christian life, for them, should be guided by the Bible as it is, "the Christian's sole rule of faith and practice" (Decker 2006:25-61). With this understanding they want to respond to HIV and AIDS guided by the biblical teaching. It is encouraging then that (as the results of this study show) there are positive readings of the Bible in Pentecostal churches for HIV response. As presented above, Pentecostals find teachings on HIV prevention, care, treatment and support in the Bible. My assessment of this turn from readings of stigmatization and discrimination to readings of care, support, treatment and identification with the infected and affected is a result of massive education programmes on HIV and AIDS. There is no substitute for education, especially education tailored along the values, culture and beliefs of the people. It is in this light that the high value occupied by the Bible in the belief system of the Pentecostals should be taken seriously in calling them to be partners to HIV and AIDS response.

Let me end this discussion by noting that biblical scholars in Africa have really played a role in demonstrating how the Bible can be used in contexts of HIV and AIDS. Musa Dube (e.g 2008), Gerald West and B. Zengele (2006), Sarojini Nadar (2004, 2007), Malebogo Kgalemang (2004), Dorothy Bea Akoto (2004), Lovemore Togarasei (2002, 2008), Madiopane Masenya (2001:186-199) and many other African scholars and theologians with interest in the Bible, have demonstrated how the Bible can be positively used by Christians for HIV and AIDS response. Unfortunately these works usually remain accessible only to the academics who rarely influence government policies and practices among the Christians who want the Bible to guide their daily lives and practices. It therefore remains a challenge to these scholars to make sure that their research findings filter down to the people who consume the Bible on a daily basis.

There is therefore need for stakeholders in national HIV and AIDS response, both governmental and non-governmental organizations, to work closely with biblical scholars in influencing the direction of biblical interpretation in churches. One way that has been promoted by the World Council of Churches' Ecumenical HIV and AIDS Initiative in Africa (EHAIA) is the mainstreaming of HIV and AIDS in biblical studies and other theological studies in theological institutions (see Dube 2003 and Chitando 2008). This helps in producing pastors trained in interpreting the Bible and theology for positive HIV and AIDS response. But there are also many other ways of encouraging the positive use of the Bible by Pentecostal churches and indeed other churches. One such other way is the conducting of workshops on biblical interpretation and HIV and AIDS.

Although time did not allow us to pursue discussions on the Bible and HIV and AIDS during the assessment workshops I have already referred to (Togarasei et al 2008), I was interested to note that participants were quite willing and enthusiastic to engage in the discussions. A number of pastors asked us if we could organize such workshops in future.

Concluding remarks

Despite the fact that it was written many years ago in a completely different world from the modern world, the Bible remains very influential in the lives of Christians, particularly those of Pentecostal churches. As we have seen, Pentecostals believe the Bible is normative and provides classic examples of how one should live a life pleasing to God. Biblical influence therefore infiltrates all aspects of a Christian's life. It is the first port of call particularly on questions to do with moral values and social responsibilities. No wonder when HIV and AIDS broke out, Christians sought answers from the Bible. In this chapter I have looked at how Pentecostal Christians in selected churches in Botswana use the Bible in contexts of HIV and AIDS. As the presentation of results of my field work shows, the Bible is used for HIV and AIDS prevention, treatment, care and support. In their response, Christians are guided by their reading of biblical texts. I have argued from an analysis of this use of the Bible that for effective involvement of Pentecostal Christians and indeed other Christians for HIV and AIDS response, the place and function of the Bible in their lives should be taken seriously.

The Christian use of the Bible should not be seen as a hindrance to effective HIV and AIDS response. What is needed, however, is to encourage a reading of the Bible that promotes effective HIV and AIDS response. This is because the meaning of the Bible is not static. In a study of the use of the Bible in the Reformed Church in Zimbabwe, L. Togarasei (2002) noted that Christians use the Bible as a classic model but allow other factors to influence their interpretation of the Bible. I found out that although the starting point for theologizing was the Bible, other factors like the church tradition and cultural practices influenced church teaching and practices. It was clear, as we have seen among Botswana Christians, that the Bible is used contextually to address modern problems that biblical people never experienced. The running of Christian hospitals, for example, was compared to Jesus' practice of healing. What Christians seek are practices comparable to those practiced in biblical times. To get to these they interpret the Bible. It is on this basis therefore that my argument that effective Christian response to HIV and AIDS should take seriously the way the Bible should be interpreted. Some of the ways of promoting this reading of the Bible have been suggested in this chapter.

Bibliography

Akoto, D. B. "Can These Bones Live? Re-reading Ezekiel 37:1-14 in the HIV/AIDS Context," in Dube, M. W. and Kanyoro, M. (eds), *Grant Me Justice!: HIV/AIDS and Gender Readings of the Bible*, Pietermaritzburg: Cluster Publications, 2004, 97-114.

Anderson, A. "Pentecostalism in Africa: an overview," *ORITA: Ibadan Journal of Religious Studies*, 36:1&2, 2004, 38-56.

Anderson, B. W. *The Living World of the Old Testament*, Essex: Longman Group UK Limited, 1993.

Asamouh-Gyadu, J. K. *African Charismatics: Current Developments within Independent Indigenous Pentecostalism in Ghana*, Leiden: Brill, 2005.

Baker, G. and Ricardo, C. "Young Men and the Construction of Masculinity in Sub-Saharan Africa: Implications for HIV/AIDS, Conflict and Violence," *The World Bank Social Development Papers: Conflict and Reconstruction Paper* No. 26, 2005.

Beasley, J. R., Fant, C. E., Joiner, E. E., Musser D. W. and Reddish, M. G. *An Introduction to the Bible,* Nashville: Abingdon Press, 1991.

Chitando, E (ed.), *Mainstreaming HIV and AIDS in Theological Education*, Geneva: WCC Publications, 2008.

Chitando, E. *Living with Hope: African Churches and HIV/AIDS 1*, Geneva: WCC Publications, 2007.

Dada, A. O. "Prosperity Gospel in Nigerian Context: A medium of social transformation or an impetus for delusion?" *ORITA: Ibadan Journal of Religious Studies*, 36:1&2, 2004, 95-105.

Dijk, R. van, ''Beyond the rivers of Ethiopia': Pentecostal pan-Africanism and Ghanaian identities in the trans-national domain," *Situating Globality:African Agency in the Appropriation of Global Culture,* W. van Binsbergen and R. van Dijk (eds.), Leiden, Boston: Brill, 2004, 171.

Decker, R.J. "Verbal –Plenary Inspiration and Translation," *Detroit Baptist Seminary Journal*, Vol. 11, 2006, 25-61.

Dube, M. W. *Postcolonial Feminist Interpretations of the Bible.* St Louis: Chalice Press, 2000.

—. (Ed.) *HIV/AIDS and the Curriculum: Methods of Integrating HIV/AIDS in Theological Programmes,* Geneva: WCC, 2003.

—. "Divining Texts for International Relations, Matthew 15:21-28," in Antonio, E P (Ed.). *Inculturation and Postcolonial Discourse in African Theology,* New York: Peter Lang, 2006, 193-208.

—. *The HIV and AIDS Bible: Selected Essays,* Scranton and London: University of Scranton Press, 2008.

Gifford, P. *African Christianity: Its Public Role,* London: Hurst and Company, 1998.

Happonen, H. "Healing in relation to HIV and AIDS," in Aaltonnen, A. et al (eds.), *Challenging the current understanding around HIV and AIDS: An African perspective,* Kenya: Starbright Services Ltd, 2005, 118-154.

Haron, M. "The Demographics of Botswana's Christian Population and BC 2001," in Nkomazana, F. and Lanner, L. (eds.), *Aspects of the History of the Church in Botswana,* Pietermaritzburg: Cluster Publications, 2007, 322-339.

Hotler, K *Yahweh in Africa: Essays on Africa and the Old Testament,* New York: Peter Lang, 2000.

Kgalemang, M. "John 9: Deconstructing the HIV/AIDS Stigma," in Dube, M. W. and Kanyoro, M. (eds), *Grant Me Justice!: HIV/AIDS and Gender Readings of the Bible,* Pietermaritzburg: Cluster Publications, 2004, 141-168.

Mabotho, T. *The Position of Pentecostal Churches on the use of condoms in the HIV and AIDS Era,* Unpublished B.A. dissertation, Department of Theology and Religious Studies, University of Botswana, 2008.

Masenya, M. "Between unjust suffering and the silent God: Job and HIV sufferers in South Africa," in *Missionalia* Vol. 29:2, 2001, 186-199.

Mbiti, J. "Do you understand what you are reading? The Bible in African homes, schools and churches," in *Missionalia* Vol.33:2, 2005, 234-248.

Mgadla, P. T. "Who used whom in the establishment of medical spheres of influence in the Bechuanaland Protectorate? The case of the Seventh Day Adventist and Moffat Hospitals in Kanye 1922-1959," in Nkomazana F. and L. Lanner (eds.), *Aspects of the history of the church in Botswana,* Pietermaritzburg: Cluster Publications, 2007, 114-159.

Munyika, V. "Confronting HIV and AIDS related stigma and its devastating consequences," in Aaltonnen, A. et al (eds.), *Challenging the current understanding around HIV and AIDS: An African perspective,* Kenya: Starbright Services Ltd, 2005, 74-117.

Nadar, S. "Module 3: Studying the Hebrew Bible in HIV and AIDS contexts," in Dube, M. W. (ed.), *HIV and AIDS Curriculum for*

Theological Education by Extension in Africa & 10 HIV and AIDS Modules, CD, Geneva: World Council of Churches, 2007.

—. "Barak God and Die!" Women, HIV and a Theology of Suffering,' in Dube , M. W. and Kanyoro, M. (eds), *Grant Me Justice!: HIV/AIDS and Gender Readings of the Bible*, Pietermaritzburg: Cluster Publications, 2004, 80-96.

Perry, S. *Responses of the Faith-Based Organisations to HIV/AIDS in Sub-Saharan Africa*, Geneva: World Council of Churches, 2003.

Stiebert, J. 'Does the Hebrew Bible have Anything to Tell us about HIV/AIDS?' in Dube, M. W. (Ed.), *HIV/AIDS and the Curriculum: Methods of Integrating HIV/AIDS in Theological Programmes,* Geneva: WCC, 2003, 24-34.

Thomas, J. C. *The Devil, Disease and Deliverance: Origins of Illness in New Testament Thought*, Sheffield: Sheffield Academic Press, 1998.

Togarasei, L. *et al, An Assessment of the Capacity of Faith-based organizations for HIV prevention in Botswana*, Gaborone: Associated Printers, 2008.

Togarasei, L. "Teaching Old Testament Studies in Zimbabwe's Theological in the HIV/AIDS era," in *Zimbabwe Journal of Educational Research* Vol. 14:3, 2002, 254-271.

—. *The Concept and Practice of Diakonia in the New Testament and its Implications in the Zimbabwean Context*, Unpublished Doctoral thesis, Harare: University of Zimbabwe, 2002.

Ugandan Monitor, *Spiritual Healing Threatening Adherence to Antiretrovirals* (www.kaisernetwork.org: accessed 17/10/08)

Ukpong, J. S. "Reading the Bible in a Global Village: Issues and Challenges from African Readings," in Ukpong, J. S. et. al. *Reading the Bible in the Global Village: Cape Town*, Atlanta: SBL, 2002, 9-40.

Weinreich, S. and Benn, C. *AIDS: Meeting the Challenge*, Geneva: WCC Publications, 2004.

West, G. and Zengele, B. "The Medicine of God: What People Living with HIV and AIDS Want (and Get) from the Bible," *Journal of Theology for Southern Africa* Vol. 125, 2006, 51-63.

PART III:

OTHER RELIGIONS

Chapter Eight

Religious NGOs and their Jihad against HIV and AIDS: The Muslim Factor in (and Beyond) Southern Africa

Muhammed Haron

Introduction

According to recent research outputs and statistics, the Third World of which Africa and Asia form an integral part appears to be the most widely infected and affected by the HIV and AIDS epidemic. This particular pandemic, which was identified in the USA in the early 1980s, has slowly made its way into the heart of the continents of Africa and Asia respectively. Since its presence on these continents, it has spread at a rapid and unstoppable pace. Its impact has thus far been detected in all spheres of human life and has forced the governments with the help of the Non-Governmental Organizations (hereafter NGOs) in general and Faith-Based Organizations (hereafter FBOs) in particular to adopt intervention strategies as a way of combating its spread and seeking solutions to stop the pandemic in its tracks. These efforts have imposed added economic and social burdens upon the governments as well as the NGOs/FBOs because the pandemic has been wreaking havoc and immeasurable hardship among communities in different parts of the Third World.

In the light of these developments, the world religious communities represented by their FBOs such as the World Council of Religion and Peace have emerged from their cloisters to help devise strategies of preventing the spread of HIV and AIDS. These FBOs have joined the ranks of secular NGOs and governments in actively combating and preventing its ongoing onslaught. Since the late 1990s FBOs have been identified as a crucial player in its prevention and have played a pivotal role in responding to their communities' needs; and they have, in fact, been in the forefront in different parts of the African continent working with professional health care workers and educationists to stem the rising tide of HIV and AIDS.

This chapter looks at the role of Muslim NGOs in their *jihad* (struggle) against HIV and AIDS in South(ern) Africa. In the first part the chapter defines, albeit briefly, FBOs; whilst this acts as an appropriate frame within which to understand the position and responses of (international) FBOs towards the HIV and AIDS pandemic, it also acts as an important backdrop to the contents of the chapter as a whole. Since the chapter makes reference to FBOs in general, it brings into view the religio-ethical principles that underpin the World Religious Systems as a whole before giving particular attention to Islam and Muslims. The chapter's second part studies the *jihad* undertaken by certain Southern African Muslim NGOs in fighting the pandemic. It intends to demonstrate the extent to which these organizations have adopted a participatory approach rather than a observatory approach in dealing with HIV and AIDS.

Conceptualizing FBOs

African nation-states, like their counterparts elsewhere in the world, consist of a variety of religious communities who are bona fide citizens of these states. These specific communities are bound together because of their common beliefs and practices. In addition, they espouse and uphold certain religious principles and strive towards the implementation of these principles in their daily lives with the objective of achieving religious salvation. These communities are not in any way 'imaginary' communities but existential ones that hold onto abstract ideals such as belief in a Supreme Being. For them, this is a vital aspect of their life in that it helps to keep them spiritually focused during their temporal earthly sojourn. However, they have constructed institutions and organizations to assist them to attain these principles and achieve their religious goals of maintaining spiritual consciousness throughout their worldly journey. These organizations, which have been identified as FBOs, have therefore been conceptualized and created to transform them to be 'one' with God or 'immersed' in God.

FBOs, which emerged from within these religious communities, have essentially been defined as 'communities of faith' that 'network' with like-minded individuals from within their communities. In the process of wanting to achieve their goals, they make use of the infrastructure that has been created by their fellow believers to further the aims of their particular religious community or order. FBOs, which are mere representatives of these communities, identify specific objectives that they wish to fulfill on behalf of or in the name of the religious community that they represent. They usually choose facilities other than their place of worship to operate from and conduct their activities. Moreover, they act as proactive agents in order to bring about socio-religious change in the behavior of the community towards issues such as HIV and AIDS. FBOs are basically religiously oriented structures, which express ideas, thoughts and practices in relation to the activity or work that is being undertaken.

Furthermore, they also choose certain approaches and adopt particular methods to achieve their religious objectives. One of the approaches that came to characterize the FBOs in their attempts to contribute effectively towards stemming the HIV and AIDS tide was becoming full participants in the process; they, in other words, consciously adopted a participatory approach that clearly demonstrated their involvement as active participants in the HIV and AIDS pandemic. They thus avoided being identified with those who preferred an observatory approach; an approach that studied and discussed the pandemic from a theoretical rather than a practical level or from a distance without getting involved with members of their congregants who have been infected and affected.

FBOs' Participatory Approach

Prior to recording the FBOs involvement in combating HIV and AIDS, we wish to provide a historical summary of the nature of the religious responses to the pandemic. The purpose for this is to observe and note the attitudinal changes that occurred over the last three decades.

Historical Phases: Religious Responses and HIV and AIDS Pandemic

When the HIV and AIDS pandemic reared its ugly head in the beginning of the 1980s, religious communities adopted an intransigent attitude towards the pandemic that was gradually making inroads among their adherents and affecting everyone (see Figure 1 below). This deafening silence on the part of the religious leadership may be attributed to their theological understanding of this pandemic's spread. As the pandemic gained momentum and when it was disclosed that it emerged within the ranks of the homosexuals, the general religious response was that HIV and AIDS was caused by the immoral, lewd, unnatural and wayward activities of this group of individuals who have been regarded as an 'accursed lot' by the extant sacred texts. The 'theologically impotent' response (Maluleke 2003:59-76) and the downright judgmental position that religious traditions held was based on the view that this was among God's signs that had come as a form of punishment (Al-Marayati 1989). Similar issues faced all other religious traditions. The question of whether it was determined by God, according to the views of the Christians and Muslims, or by some power, according to the understanding of the Buddhists, has been a debatable point amongst the theologians and religious educators. The theological questions raised by the 2000 WCC Study document are also applicable to the Muslims (WCC 2000). This cold-shouldered approach was prevalent throughout the 'Denial Phase' that stretched from the 1980s until beyond 1993. It may be argued that throughout this period the religious leadership and FBOs adopted an obscurantist, dogmatic and self-righteous position that did not help the plight of those who had been infected and affected (see Figure 2 below).

However, with the passage of time and as statistics were made available that demonstrated the rapid increase in the number of PLWHA from among the religious communities, the religious leadership and activists found it difficult to adhere to their obstinate stance towards this pandemic. This thus resulted in the adoption of a slightly different position. They realized along with many NGOs that they had to break the silence because the disease was having a detrimental effect on the lives of many in their communities and that there was a need to assist in educating their congregational members of its traumatic consequences. Their response thus ushered in what may be described as the 'Breaking the Silence Phase' (Cassiem 2002), a phase that started in 1994 and continued until 1999 with the formation of FBOs on the local, national and international levels.

A new phase began when a growing number of FBOs were co-opted by governments and brought on board by international NGOs that were very aware of the potential force that exist within the hands of the religious leaders and their communities. This formed part of what may be called the 'Acknowledgement Phase;' this coincided with the closing of the 20th century and the beginning of the 21st century. Since 1999 many FBOs have cooperated with secular NGOs and their governments and this has resulted in the recording of many success stories in a few African states.

Figure 1: Historical Phases of religious responses to HIV and AIDS (from Cassiem 2002)

Religious Responses towards HIV/Aids: Historical Phases

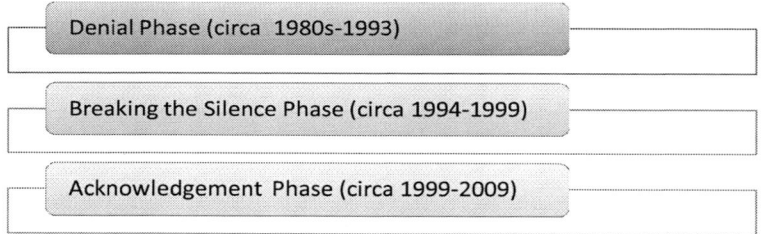

Denial Phase (circa 1980s-1993)

Breaking the Silence Phase (circa 1994-1999)

Acknowledgement Phase (circa 1999-2009)

a) International FBO participation

Throughout the 'acknowledgment phase' important international religious bodies and organizations have placed HIV and AIDS on their agendas as part of their strategy to assist governments and international NGOs to deal with the pandemic. The Chicago based Parliament of World Religions (www.cpwr.org est. 1893) and the New York based World Council of Religion and Peace (www.wcrp.org est. 1961) are two international religious bodies that have adopted proactive positions on the issue. At the '15th International AIDS Conference in Bangkok, Thailand: Religious Leaders convene to combat HIV/AIDS Related Stigma,' which took place during the month of July 2004, members of these bodies actively participated and shared their thoughts on how to address the pandemic. In addition to these bodies, other well known international NGOs such as World Vision (www.worldvision.org) developed creative projects to deal with the scourge; for example, it set up the 'Hope for African Children Initiative' (cf. www.hopeforafricanchildren.org) that forms part of World Vision's general activities and demonstrates concretely its concerns in combating the spread of HIV and AIDS among children who are indeed a very vulnerable group in society.

Figure 2: FBO Responses

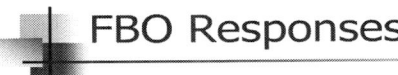

FBO Responses

- Theologically Impotent
- Obstructionist
- Close-minded
- Dogmatic
- Extremist
- Judgmental
- Self-righteous
- COLD-SHOULDER Approach

- Theologically Virile
- Cooperative
- Open-minded
- Pragmatic
- Liberal
- Non-Judgmental
- Selfless
- WARM-HEARTED Approach

Prior to 1999 many international institutions such as Family Health International (www.fhi.org.uk) have raised concerns regarding the absence of the religious organizations in participating in preventing the spread of HIV and AIDS. When they planned for their 11th International Conference on AIDS and STDs in Africa which took place in Lusaka in 1999, representatives of FBOs were invited with the objective of making an effective input in this area. It was then that they set up the Africa Forum of FBOs in Reproductive Health with the aim of promoting dialogue on ethical and moral issues that have until then been acting as barriers to the FBOs participation. This was followed in June 2000 with the formation of the Global Interfaith Alliance (www.thegaia.org) to combat HIV and AIDS and soon thereafter, USAID also mooted the idea of CORE Communities (cf. Shuaibu 2002).

b) HIV and AIDS and its impact on FBOs

The increasing participation of FBOs in the health care sector with the specific objective of addressing HIV and AIDS has resulted, at least, in many positive outcomes. The first is that the HIV and AIDS pandemic have been instrumental in bringing diverse religious organizations together to seek strategies of addressing it. This has indirectly contributed towards the formation of a vibrant religious pluralist environment and a way of defusing the influence of religious fundamentalist groups in international affairs. Although it might be unlikely that the latter voices will disappear, the religious developments do give a positive spin to inter-religious dialogue and cooperation.

The second spin-off of this HIV and AIDS pandemic is that it encouraged religious communities to re-dedicate themselves to upholding religious values by being loyal and faithful to their families, neighbors, societies and their nation-state. This dedication and devotion have been stressed in the light of the pandemic having taken away individuals from all and sundry and without distinguishing between rich and poor families or the rural and urban communities. And a third outcome of this pandemic is that it has demanded religious communities to be doubly committed. On the one hand, they commit themselves to protect their societies from being infected and affected, and on the other, they commit themselves to work with (secular) NGOs in both the educational and health care sectors to disseminate relevant information about the epidemic with the hope of eradicating its spread.

Since FBOs have employed their religious assets such as their respective religions' ethical teachings to guide the contemporary society in order to adopt a moral and healthy lifestyle that is in tune with the divine commands, the UN has recognized and acknowledged the importance of religion when it organized the '1st International Conference on AIDS and Religion' in Dakar (Senegal) in 1998 (cf. www.unaids.org). At the 'UNGASS First Informal Consultation Meeting,' which was held towards the end of February in New York 2001, the FBOs statement highlighted the specific strengths the FBOs possessed in mobilizing themselves against the HIV and AIDS pandemic. According to this public statement, the FBOs had the 'reach, experience/capacity, spiritual mandate and sustainability' to effectively deal with the pandemic (cf. www.hnet.org/UNGASS%20docs/UNGASS%20Infl/Faith%20Based%Organizations.ht ml). At another meeting facilitated by the World Council of Churches for the UN Special General Assembly on HIV and AIDS during June 2001, it was firmly argued for 'Increased Partnership between FBOs, Governments and Inter-Government Organizations' (cf. www.wcc-coe.org/wcc/what /mission/ny-statement.html).

On this point, scholars such as E. Green (2002) and J. Liebowitz (2002) have cogently argued in favor of the FBOs participation in helping to reduce HIV transmission. Both observed that ample data and solid evidence have been produced. Their papers showed that FBOs have a 'significant' and 'comparative advantage' in promoting 'primary behavior change.' Green, as a matter of fact, hypothesized that this type of behavior change might be among the most effective interventions if FBOs are given the opportunity to share their rich, spiritual assets. He also emphasized that FBOs should be supported in their efforts to promote abstinence and fidelity. Elsewhere Green (2003) pointed out that FBOs were the major providers of care and support services to their respective communities and were uniquely positioned to disseminate HIV and AIDS education and prevention messages through their extensive religious networks that connect cities, towns and villages in the remotest parts of their countries.

Green (2002) further demonstrated through case studies the positive role Christian FBOs such as World Vision, The Salvation Army, and Catholic Relief Services have played and the innovative programs that they thus implemented to contain the pandemic. At a three-day HIV and AIDS workshop for FBOs and National AIDS Councils of five African states in Addis Ababa during May 2003 the Patriarch of the Ethiopian Orthodox Church, Abune Paulos, echoed the view that is generally held by all, that the religious beliefs are deeply embedded in African societies and that their FBOs have the opportunity to exercise tremendous moral authority to influence the lifestyle of individuals and bring about behavioral change. He stated that "religious organizations have a primary responsibility to save lives. They are entrusted by God not only to save souls but also to care and foster for the well being of man" (Anon 2003). Taking into account the critical statement of the Patriarch of the Ethiopian Orthodox Church, it is perhaps instructive to turn our attention at this stage in the essay to some of the religio-ethical principles that have been disseminated by most – if not all – religious traditions in and outside the African continent.

Religio-Ethical Principles

Now that sufficient reference has been made to the participation of FBOs in the educational and social-health sectors to fight the epidemic, it would be appropriate to shift focus to the religious-ethical principles that underpin their philosophies. However, since it will be beyond the scope of this essay to deal with all the religious traditions, the essay will only make reference to Buddhism and Islam. But in order to have an insight into these two traditions' religio-ethical teachings, general reference will have to be made to the other religious traditions. Three of the religious precepts in the respective Judeo-Christian and Buddhist traditions have been captured in Figure 3 to comprehend some of the ideas that underpin the behaviour patterns of the followers of these traditions. Since Islam is usually associated with Judaism and Christianity, it is not surprising to have found that Islam brought into its religio-ethical system the Judeo-Christian Ten Commandments, and that Taoism absorbed some of the Buddhist ethical teachings. From these examples, it is quite clear that ethical teachings have been inherited by certain traditions and passed on to others; whilst some

faded away, others have continued and remained indisputably common to
the major and minor religious traditions.

Figure 3: Select Religio-Ethical Principles

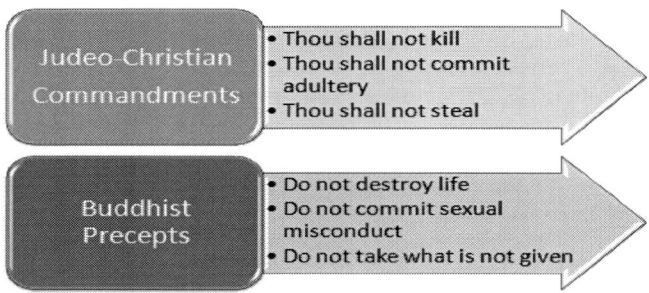

At this juncture it might be useful to briefly define what is meant by
'religious ethical teachings.' According to scholarly musings on the
subject, religious ethics "includes all the sacred norms that inform
ordinary behavior" and it forms an important dimension of religion, which
is a vital aspect of human experience (Chidester 1987). It is an accepted
fact that ethical norms – standards, guidelines, rules, regulations, laws, and
values – are interwoven with all other aspects of belief, action and
experience that make up a religious tradition (Chidester 1987). When we
peruse Hinduism, Buddhism and Taosim, we note the common ethical
strands that permeate these traditions and the same accounts for Judaism,
Christianity and Islam. In fact, a closer study of all of these religious
traditions demonstrates that the ethical teachings embedded in and
disseminated by the monotheistic religions, on the one hand, and in the
non-monotheistic religions are not very different from one another.

Since all of these traditions share these common ethical strands, many
have emphasized these as a basis for forging inter-religious co-operation
and dialogue in the HIV and AIDS arena. Within this era of globalization,
whilst the differences that exist amongst each of these traditions are well
known and accepted, there has also been the acknowledgment of the
common connection that is prevalent and which should be fully exploited
in the interest of all religious communities and without any form of
discrimination. The Biblical command: 'Thou shall not commit adultery'

within the Judeo-Christian and Islamic traditions ties in well with 'Do not commit sexual misconduct' found within the Buddhist-Taoist traditions.

Both groups, the monotheists (Jews, Christians and Muslims) and non-monotheists (Hindus, Buddhists and Taoists) have reinforced this particular ethical command within the wider ethical system which their theologians developed, implemented and strictly enforced over the many generations. In this regard, it must however be observed that "religious ethics does not simply constitute of sets of instructions for what to do and what not to do; (and) it is not simply a code of injunctions and prohibitions; religious ethics involves a more dynamic pattern of behaviour in relating to the sacred norms .... it consists of not only standards for everyday, ordinary behavior, but also a variety of human responses to these standards" (Chidester 1987:53). Bearing this comment in mind, one should therefore understand these commands or injunctions within their contexts as well as fully comprehend their local and universal implications; this should be particularly so in the contemporary world, where human rights activists would argue against the punishment of adulterers as enjoined by the Biblical and Quranic texts respectively. That aside, let us use the Muslims as a case study to demonstrate how they have undertaken *jihad* (struggle) against HIV and AIDS within the Southern African region. However, since this is a vast region, specific examples will be drawn from certain Southern African countries.

Muslims Organizations and their 'Jihad' against HIV and AIDS

The Muslim heartlands are located in the Northern African, South West Asian and South East Asian parts of the world map. However, during the latter part of the 20th century many of its adherents have shifted to Europe and the Americas where they have formed sizeable numbers. Many of them have lived in Southern Africa for a number of generations and this has resulted in them being bona fide citizens of the nation-states that make up this important region. Before we show how they have addressed the HIV and AIDS pandemic in the region, we wish to briefly provide an insight into their beliefs and lifestyle.

a) Muslims: Their Basic Beliefs and Lifestyle

Islam has been and is still described as a religion of peace and salvation (Rahman 1979). Whilst it has absorbed some of the traditions and teachings of the other monotheistic traditions as already mentioned, it charted out its unique features that make it distinct from them. Like the Buddhist teachings, it also harps on the 'mean path' or the 'middle road' that would lead to the road to the truth and ultimate salvation.

Muhammad, whom the Muslims believe as God's final messenger after having sent all the previous ones such as Moses and Jesus, is regarded as their exemplar and model. He was the one, according to their historical sources, who was the recipient of God's revelation – known as the Quran, the primary source of Islam – and its sole commentator, and thus showed the way through his words and deeds. He thus expounded upon and explained the belief system and five pillars of Islam, which in turn contained its ethical teachings. For example, when addressing 'sex' as a topic it will be observed that it forms part of 'moral education' - a section which follows the chapter on 'cleanliness' in the jurisprudential texts – and is not offered as a separate unrelated subject but as an outcome of following religio-ethical principles enshrined in the Quran and practices of Muhammad (Dar 1999). This method is based upon the notion that the person's spiritual life and physical existence are inextricably tied and that the one has an effect on the other. Muhammad's central role in the establishment and dissemination of an Islamic lifestyle implied that his statements and acts were and are crucial for the Muslim to heed. One such prophetic statement that may be applied to those infected by HIV and AIDS is: "Whoever does the needful for his/her brother/sister, God does the needful for him. Whoever removes distress of one who submits (to God), God removes for him/her distress ..." and in another: "God has no mercy on him/her who is not merciful to humankind"(Ali 1983: 386). These statements clearly demonstrate that the Muslim has a social obligation towards his/her fellow human beings.

Bearing these thoughts in mind, it should also be remembered that Muslims have been enjoined to perform the daily ritual prayers as a way of cultivating themselves spiritually through constant communication with God, and with the sincere hope of achieving salvation. However, the enactment of these daily prayers - as well as the other pillars such as fasting and the giving of the purificatory text to the poor and needy - is not sufficient for the attainment of salvation. The individual is expected to also perform other duties such as caring for the orphan, the sick, the needy and the wayfarer. The social dimension and duties are, in a sense, obligatory because one has to be concerned about one's family members, neighbor, community and nation. Since HIV and AIDS affected large parts of the society, a Muslim is expected to extend a helping hand and assist those that have been infected and those that have been affected.

In the light of these teachings, a Muslim should abstain from and avoid an unhealthy lifestyle. This entails keeping away from the types of foods (e.g. pork) Islam forbade them to consume, and it implies that they should steer clear of indulging in sexual relationships outside wedlock; in other words, consuming forbidden foods and engaging in adulterous relationships are viewed as harmful at both the individual/familial and social levels. The individual and community should therefore try to avoid indulging in these activities and cultivate a lifestyle that harmonizes with the rest of his/her society according to God's injunctions.

The Muslim individual is encouraged to pray and ask God for good in this life and in the Hereafter, and that "no supplication is more pleasing to God than a request for good health" (cf. www.positivemuslims.org and see also, Fakir 1978: 31-33 & 400-402). These tie in with the view that in order to live a good and healthy life one should get to know what is beneficial and what is harmful; and this can only be attained through becoming knowledgeable about one's body, one's environment, and one's society. There is another statement attributed to Muhammad, which reads: "The seeking of knowledge is obligatory upon everyone who submits (to God)" (Ali 1983: 39). This statement thus encouraged individuals to pursue all sorts of knowledge and information that will be of benefit not only to oneself but to all human beings. Armed with the knowledge of the beneficial and the harmful, good and bad, right and wrong, one should be able to assist in affirming one's belief in God and faithfully follow the ethical rules that were set down by Him in the sacred texts such as the Bible and the Quran. If a Muslim transgresses God's injunctions and disregards the basic social duties then he/she has not heeded the ethical teachings of Islam and is thus liable for his/her actions on the day of Resurrection when each and everyone will account for his/her actions during their temporal, earthly sojourn. This can be gauged from the prophetic statements quoted above.

Since Muslims are, on the one hand, expected to perform the obligatory rituals that help to purify them, they are, on the other, also expected to serve society in which ever manner they possibly can. This approach, which is distinctly participatory – an approach that was mentioned earlier, has been adopted by Muslim NGOs that have dedicated themselves to work with individuals that have been infected and also with communities that have been affected.

b) Muslim NGOs in Southern Africa and Beyond

In the last 15 years (circa 1995-2010) many Muslim NGOs were established in different parts of Southern African with the intention of tackling various issues in the development sector. Despite the existence of HIV and AIDS, there was no dedicated Muslim NGO that targeted the vulnerable groups in the Southern African region. Nonetheless, as the presence of the pandemic became more pronounced and as it affected religious communities, groups of concerned Muslims initiated the idea of creating a forum that gave its full attention to those infected and affected by this pandemic. In South Africa one organization that had been established to solely address the HIV and AIDS problem was Positive Muslims (Ahmed 2003) and the Muslim NGO that gave its attention to it though it began as a professional health care organization, was the Islamic Medical Association of Uganda; a professional medical association outside the Southern African region. Let us begin and provide pen portraits of these and other organizations and their concomitant programs and activities in trying to arrest the spread of HIV and AIDS.

Figure 4: Muslim NGOs: their Projects and Programmes

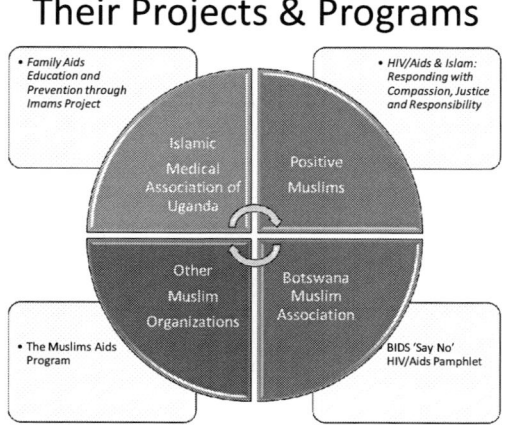

Islamic Medical Association of Uganda (IMAU)

The IMAU, which modeled itself on the South African Islamic Medical Association (hereafter IMASA), was established by Muslim health professionals in 1988. It aimed at effectively contributing towards the health-sector in Uganda. As early as 1989, when IMAU became aware of the pandemic, they organized a National Workshop for Muslim Qadi (judges) and AIDS education training programs for Imams. Their early confrontation with and experience of the HIV and AIDS pandemic triggered an automatic response and that was how the IMAU as professional health care workers can make a substantial input that would assisting in arresting the HIV and AIDS pandemic's continuous advance among Uganda's vulnerable communities. Since they realized that it needed team work they consciously decided to collaborate in 1992 with Multi-Sectoral Aids Control Approach (MACA) that was Uganda's AIDS control program.

As already indicated, from the very start the IMAU was quite prepared to see how it could effectively halt the onslaught of the pandemic. Even though it was prepared to provide the necessary medical assistance, it deliberately targeted the Imams who were the most influential group within the Ugandan Muslim society. Fortunately for IMAU these trained theologians, who were the appointed religious leaders of the Muslims, were quite willing to participate in whatever IMAU had to offer. This attitude lightened IMAU's burden and it eased their task in carrying out their plans to tackle the scourge.

Over a five year period from 1992 until 1997, IMAU not only trained Imams around the country but also a sizeable number of volunteers (approximately 7,000). Their mobilization of volunteers and the educational programs increased the Muslim community's awareness and knowledge threefold and this resulted in a rapid decrease in the number of individuals who were affected and became infected. In fact, the IMAU's *Family AIDS Education and Prevention through Imams Project* succeeded in spreading accurate knowledge about HIV and AIDS prevention, bringing about positive behavior change regarding safer sex methods, and educating the communities about the gender-adolescent relations and constant counseling. IMAU also initiated the *Madrasa AIDS Education and Prevention Project* that devised appropriate graded syllabi and curricula; the curriculum included lessons that focused, inter alia, on healthy living, understanding sexuality from the Muslim perspective, breaking the stigma and adopting safer sex methods.

IMAU's techniques and contributions towards HIV and AIDS prevention in Uganda in particular and the region in general have been recorded as an important success story that has been enlisted by UNAIDS researchers and

scholars as a significant 'best practice;' this has been published online at
www.unaids.org/publications/documents/sectors/religion/imamscse.pdf
with the hope that many in and beyond the region would derive lessons
from the innovative Ugandan experiment.

Positive Muslims: A Muslim FBO

Positive Muslims (hereafter PM [www.positivemuslims.org.za]) was set
up in 2000 by Dr. Farid Esack – who was then a member of South Africa's
Commission for Gender Equality and currently Professor at the University
of Johannesburg, Abdul-Kayyum Ahmed – an HIV and AIDS researcher
and worker, and Ms. Faghmeda Millar – a Cape Town Muslim woman that
was HIV positive and who has worked tirelessly with other FBOs such as
IMASA that have also been active on this front. Though PM had little
support at the outset, they persevered and slowly convinced individuals
and groups through various seminars, workshops, public lectures and radio
interviews about the HIV and AIDS scourge and how the community
cannot afford to turn a blind eye towards the realities surrounding them.

The organization focused on three areas:

- Creating awareness and educating the community through seminars
  and working with HIV positive persons;
- Supporting positive persons, giving counseling to their affected
  families and providing skills training; and
- Engaging in research and monitoring the Muslim responses to the
  pandemic.

PM has been successfully hosting various programs and have also been
pamphleteering and putting up posters as a method of disseminating
information. It also has a newsletter with the same title in which it shares
information as to what the organization has accomplished and other related
information. Dr. Esack, who has been the driving force behind PM from
the outset, edited a 'Theology of Compassion' publication titled *HIV/AIDS
& Islam: Responding with Compassion, Justice and Responsibility* that
provided salient ideas as regards the general Muslim response. It offered a
fair insight as to how the pandemic should be understood within the
Islamic context, and it showed how Muslims should respect God's
boundaries through taking charge of their lives, and the tackling of the
epidemic head-on. And as a follow to his earlier work, he co-edited with S.
Chiddy *Islam and AIDS: Between Scorn, Pity and Justice* that brought

together serious scholarly reflections on HIV and AIDS among Muslims (Haron 2010).

Botswana Muslim Association (BMA) HIV and AIDS Programme

BMA is the parent body that oversees all Muslims activities in Botswana. For the past number of years it has been chaired by Mr. Abul-Sattar Dada who is one of Gaborone's well-known business figures. Under his leadership BMA was able to make its mark in various sectors of Botswana. Nevertheless, the BMA continues to be active in the social, cultural and political arenas and has many important affiliates. One of these affiliates is the Gaborone Mosque Committee that takes charge of all mosque affairs from providing education to the learners to the collection of the annual purificatory tax. Another important affiliate is the Botswana Islamic Da'wah Society (hereafter BIDS) that has been under the leadership of Shaykh Hassan, a Burundian born theologian who has been in Botswana for close to 15 years.

It is this organization that devised and implemented an HIV and AIDS program. Although BIDS has not been as proactive as IMAU and PM, it has been actively monitoring to what extent Muslims have been infected and affected by HIV and AIDS. However, one area which they have effectively used is that of pamphleteering about the prevention of HIV and AIDS. They issued a one page pamphlet that identifies what is HIV and what is AIDS. In addition, it also briefly explains how it is not transmitted and the actual truth about sex and HIV. The BIDS pamphlet stressed that 'fear of God is the best way to protect yourself and others from HIV and AIDS and seem to hold the position that relationships outside marriage (i.e. adultery) have been one of the contributory factors of the spread of HIV.

The front cover of the light-blue pamphlet contains an oft-quoted Quranic verse (chapter 3 verse 110) and an interestingly (upside down) HIV and AIDS symbol. The symbol was deliberately constructed in this manner because it coincides with the Arabic word for 'no' (transliterated as 'la') and the English words 'say no' overlay the symbol. Below the symbol, there are five bullets that declare: Say no: (i) to sex before marriage, (ii) to pre-marital courtship (iii) to alcohol, (iv) to drugs and (v) to HIV and AIDS. According to the available statistics on those infected, there have been no known cases among the small Muslim community. If there, however, are cases then it appears that the infected individuals have opted to remain silent instead of publicizing their cases.

On the whole BIDS have been influenced by the programs that have been devised and adopted in South Africa. In fact, BMA has generally been dependent on the views of the South African Muslim theological bodies (eg. Jamiatul Ulama [i.e. a body of Muslim Theological Body in Gauteng]) on HIV and AIDS and other theological matters. The BMA would not commit itself to a project unless the Gauteng theologians gave the go ahead. Let us end off by looking at other organizations in South Africa that have devoted their energies in combating HIV and AIDS in the northern part of South Africa.

Other Muslim NGOs

Positive Muslims' methods stimulated other FBOs in South Africa to also adopt and adapt their ideas. These Muslim FBOs, namely the Islamic Careline, IMASA and the Jamiatul Ulama, have implemented a specially designed 'The Muslim AIDS Program' that differs slightly from the PM program. In their joint pamphlet they talked about the social evils that have been vehemently condemned in Islam, namely adultery, homosexuality and the consumption of intoxicants. As far as they are concerned, the HIV and AIDS issue is a social and moral problem, and, according to them, HIV and AIDS' root cause is as a result of immoral sexual behavior, and it is this behavior that must be rectified and radically changed.

Instead of supporting the idea of 'Safe sex' (distributed as stickers), they have been popularizing the idea of 'Save sex' (until one is married); and came out with another sticker, which read: 'Faithful sex' and not 'Fateful sex.' This slogan also highlighted the view that sex should be performed faithfully within the institution of marriage and not outside it, which amounts to 'fateful sex.' On one of their bookmarkers they have a message to the youth and with an apt slogan: Be Wise ... Moralise! (cf. www.islamsa.org.za). In yet another slogan the words were slightly amended; instead of reading: Abstinence, Be Faithful, Condomize, it read: Abstinence, Be Faithful and Take Care. In this instance, it once again demonstrated that there has been no approval from within the Muslim NGO sector of accepting a condomizing approach; this, they have argued, gives license to illicit sex which is not acceptable within the Islamic ethical system.

Conclusion

In concluding this chapter, it should be mentioned that all these religious communities have worked towards dispelling the fear and stigma associated with the pandemic. In addition, they have also actively educated their communities about being gender sensitive, about the significance of informing the young adolescents about the positive aspects of 'sex' that forms an integral part of human life and to re-look at the respective positions of culture and religion within contemporary society. This meant that the theologians, religious teachers, cultural educators and a host of others have had to deal with a number of issues that were taboo a few years or a number of generations ago, and discuss the issue in the public media and in private forums, and more particularly in the households and religious schools. Although many have still not accepted this new form of education and the methods that have been adopted, inroads were made in many sectors of society and one assumes that this will continue to be part of the road towards finding a solution to the pandemic.

As stated earlier in the essay, all religious traditions share certain ethical principles that are accepted as part of their belief systems and practiced on a daily basis. These common principles are the ones that need to be highlighted and employed to foster better human relationships particularly in the fight against the pandemic. It has been demonstrated that where FBOs have worked together, successful results have been forthcoming, where the work has been half-heartedly implemented by insincere and non-committed FBOs, the patients and supporting families have suffered tremendously.

FBOs have and will continue to play a positive and dynamic role in the prevention of HIV and AIDS. However, they will need to continuously draw sustenance and guidance from their sacred texts in order to make a significant change in the societies they serve. They have to show that they sincerely care for those who are suffering from and affected by the epidemic, and they should demonstrate through dedication and commitment that they are prepared to work with the non-religious sector specially the health sector to find a solution and a cure for the epidemic. Even though there have been success stories in certain countries such as Uganda, African governments and their partners in the NGO sector such as the FBOs, cannot afford to rest on their laurels and allow HIV and AIDS to claim lives and wreak havoc with state economies, health systems and social structures; they need to be armed with hope and dedication, the relevant knowledge to stem the HIV and AIDS tide and make a qualitative difference.

Bibliography

Ahmed, A. K. Developing a Theology of Compassion: Muslim attitudes towards people living with HIV/AIDS in South Africa. *Annual Review of Islam in South Africa,* 3: 22-26, December 2000.
—. *Positive Muslims: A Critical Analysis of Muslims Aids activism in relation to women living with HIV/AIDS in Cape Town.* Unpublished MA Anthropology & Sociology Thesis: University of the Western Cape, 2003.
Ali, M. *A Manuel of Hadith.* London: Curzon, 1983.
Al-Maryati, A. Islam Aids: A Sign of God? In G. Melton (ed.), *The Churches Speak on Aids: Official Statements from Religious Bodies and Ecumenical Organizations,* Detroit: Gale Research, 1989 , 178-182.
Anon. *The Muslim Child in the Battle against HIV/Aids.* Wellington: Adab Islamic Welfare Association, 2001.
Anon. *Faith-Based Organization should play unique role in fight against AIDS: Patriach.* (Text: http://www.waltainfo.com/EnNews/2003/May/14May03/may14e4.htm), 2003.
Bukusi, E. Breaking the Shell of Silence. *Forum Review: Religious Organizations and Productive Health.* No. 2 July 2000.
Campbell, D. and Rader, A. *HIV/Aids, Stigma and Religious Responses: An Overview of Issues Relating to Stigma and the Religious Sector in Africa.* (full text: www.ccih.org/compendium/HIV-AIDS. 2001).
Cassiem, A. *The Muslims' Response to HIV/Aids.* Cape Town: Social Development Unit - University of the Western Cape, 2002.
Chidester, D. *Patterns of Action: Religion and Ethics in Comparative Perspective.* Belmont, Ca.: Wadsworth Publishing, 1987.
Conze, E. *Buddhism: Its Essence and Development.* New Delhi: Munshiram Manoharlal, 1994.
Dar, B. A. "Ethical Teachings of the Quran" in M.M. Sharif's (ed) *A History of Muslim Philosophy.* Delhi: Low Price Publications, Vol. 1 ch. 8, repr. 1999.
Dube, M. W. (ed). *HIV/Aids and the Curriculum: Methods of Integrating HIV/Aids in Theological Programmes.* Geneva: WCC, 2004.
Esack, F. *HIV/AIDS & Islam: Responding with Compassion, Justice and Responsibility.* Cape Town: Positive Muslims, 2004.
Esack. F. & Chiddy, S (eds). *Islam and AIDS: Between Scorn, Pity and Justice.* Oxford: Oneworld, 2009.
Fakier, A. *Manual of Prayer and Fasting.* Cape Town: Al-Jamia Institute of Islamic Studies, 1978.

Green, E. *Abstinence, Fidelity and the Contribution of Religious Communities to Reduce HIV Transmission.* School of Public Health: Harvard University, November 2002.

Green, E. *Faith-Based Organizations: Contributions to HIV Prevention.* School of Public Health: Harvard University, September, 2003.

Haron, M. A Book Review of F. Esack & S. Chiddy's (eds.) *Islam and AIDS: Between Scorn, Pity and Justice* (Oxford: Oneworld 2009) in *SAHARA: Journal of Social Aspects of HIV/Aids* 7(1): 94-95, July 2010. Online: www.sahara.com, 2010.

Jackson, H. *Aids Africa: Continent in Crisis.* Southern Africa HIV/AIDS Harare: Information Dissemination Services, 2002.

Liebowitz, J. *Are Faith-Based Organizations Uniquely Placed to Counteract HIV/AIDS Epidemic?* Durban: Health, Economics & HIV/Aids Research Division - University of KwaZulu Natal. (Full text: www.eldis.org/static/DOC11101.htm), 2002.

—. *The Impact of Faith-Based Organizations on HIV/Aids Prevention and Mitigation in Africa.* (Full text: www.nu.ac.za/heard/papers/2002/ FBOs%20paper_Dec02.pdf), 2002.

Mohamed, A. An Overview of the social ills and the spectre of HIV/AIDS amongst Muslims in the Cape. *Journal of the Islamic Medical Association,* 1997.

Maluleke, T. "Towards an HIV/Aids sensitive curriculum" in Musa Dube's (ed.) *HIV/AIDS and the Curriculum: Methods of Integrating HI/AIDS in Theological Programs.* Geneva: WCC, 2003.

Pyne-Mercier, L. *HIV/AIDS Prevention, Care and Support across Faith-Based Communities.* Durham, NC: Family Health International. (full text: ww.fhi.org), 2004.

Rahman, F. *Islam.* Chicago: Chicago University Press, 1979.

Shuiabu, M. *Africa Forum of FBOs in Reproductive Health and HIV/AIDS.* AF-AIDS. (Full text: http://archives.healthdev.net/af-aids), 2002.

World Council of Churches. *Facing AIDS: Study Document and Statement on HIV/AIDS*, Geneva: WCC, 2000.

—. *Facing Aids: The Challenge, the Churches' Response.* Geneva: WCC, 2002.

CHAPTER NINE

THE FAITH OF OUR FATHERS:
COLLABORATING WITH TRADITIONAL
HEALERS IN HIV AND AIDS RESPONSE

KIPTON E. JENSEN AND LEILA KATIRAYI

Public health programs in developing countries -- and among minorities or foreign-born groups within developed countries -- would be more effective if those who design and implement programs possessed an empirically based understanding of existing ethnomedical beliefs and practices and designed and implemented programs with these in mind (Green 1999: 217-218; also Airhihebuwa 1991).

Introduction

As the HIV and AIDS crisis shows no sign of slowing in Botswana, it becomes necessary to examine other approaches and perhaps overlooked opportunities. Botswana is rich in culture and traditional beliefs, beliefs that shape and influence Batswana behavior. At the center of traditional thought and belief systems is the traditional healer, the interpreter who advises the Batswana on a range of matters. Traditional healers are currently not recognized by the Ministry of Health as a form of health care delivery but remain a source of health care delivery for many in Botswana. They, however, have access to a large part of the population who may not access health care clinics. Previous researches have shown that traditional healers in sub-Saharan Africa are interested in collaboration, but few studies explore the challenges preventing collaboration. The chapter explores the challenges to collaboration between traditional healers and allopathic practitioners in Botswana and to understand Tswana conceptualization of HIV and AIDS. The findings are based on interviews with traditional healers and key informants in Botswana.

Traditional healers in Botswana

In Botswana, there are two primary traditional healing guilds: *Botswana Dingaka Association* and the *Dingaka Tsa Setso*, both of which extend in membership across the nation and both of which claim membership of approximately 1,500. These professional networks do not extend, however, to numerous traditional village healers who have not elected to belong to neither association but whom are credible in their own right on the basis of regional authority. In addition to the Batswana traditional healers there is also a strong constituency of healers from other African countries such as South Africa, Malawi, Zimbabwe, Mozambique, Ghana, etc. There is a government-sponsored HIV and AIDS Awareness Action Group for Traditional Healers – namely, *Bathusi* [literally, the Helpers].

Even within the realm of traditional healers, the mode of treatment and intervention is varied. "Though within most nations there are usually a large number of medical sub-cultures, each with its own characteristics and structure," suggests Murray Last, "policy-makers often have in mind apparently a single, paradigmatic culture from which they generalize about 'traditional medicine'" (1986: 4). This is probably still true, twenty-five years later, of most international if not also national HIV and AIDS policy-makers and public health officials in Botswana. Botswana certainly contains complex herbal traditions mixed with variant forms of divination. The majority of traditional or indigenous healers (*Dingaka tsa Setso*) involved in HIV treatment in Mogoditshane (site of study as explained under 'Methods' below) identified themselves as Herbalists (*Dingaka e tshotshwa*), Diviner-Healers (e.g., *Dingaka tsa ditaola*), Sangomas (Ancestor Intercession) or Spiritual Healers (*Moporofeta/ Moapostola*).

In terms of divination methods, most traditional healers are considered to be ritual experts or someone specially gifted to communicate with the spirits, gain answers and provide treatments for illnesses. Some traditional herbalists, and most neo-herbalists, rely solely on verbal consultation to prescribe the best herbal remedy. There are two very helpful Setswana terms for describing healing. Traditional healers make a distinction between treating and curing: *go ritibatsa* refers to the alleviation of the symptoms of a specific affliction; *go alafa* , on the other hand, means 'to cure or heal' the root cause of the affliction. *Go alefa* practices aim at comprehending and reversing the affliction. *Go thaya* ritual practices (e.g., *go thaya motse* or *go bapola lefatse*), affirm or renew the orderly structure of the social world itself (see Camaroff, 1985: 84 ff.). Methods of divination among *Dingaka tsa Setso* can include instruments such as mirrors, sacred bones and divining tablets (*ditaola*). The title "*ngaka ya ditaola,"* for example, refers to a traditional herbalist or healer who uses divining tablets to diagnose the cause and meaning of the affliction as well as to prescribe the appropriate treatment. By way of contrast to *Dingaka* and *Sangomas*, the *Moporofeti* (healer-prophet) is said to derive his or her healing powers from the Holy Spirit.

The role of the traditional healer in Africa, at least traditionally, extended well beyond their expertise in preventing and treating or curing various ailments. They were also essential in their role as advisors to the *kgosi* (chief), as intermediaries between the here-and-now and the yonder-realm of *badimo* (ancestors) and as facilitators of the stability of the local community (Neumann and Lauro, 1982).

Studies suggest that patients in southern Africa often consult traditional healers before visiting allopathic doctors and that they also rely on the counsel and advice of the former when it comes to the interpretation of the disease (Benn 2002: 9). As care providers of first resort, traditional healers are not only consulted for medical problems but social issues such as marriage problems, looking for a spouse, finding a job, familial problems, jealousy, fears, and other needs. They provide guidance and counseling to their patients. According to UNAIDS, "[t]raditional healers provide client-centered, personalized health care that is culturally appropriate, holistic and focused on meeting the needs of the individual patient" (2000: 10). The traditional healer offers more than just a cure for an ailment; the healer provides a rationale for why such an ailment has occurred. In Setswana culture, patients often want to know *why* an ailment has occurred. Traditional healers offer such explanations which are often based on moral infractions. As Heald says:

> Even if remedies are sought from the modern sector, one might surmise that the reasons for many are still sought in the indigenous one...The remedies offered by biomedicine are unlikely to be seen as absolute cures, which can be achieved only through more direct and active attempts to counter the source of the misfortune...With AIDS the adequacy of biomedicine fails not just in its lack of a satisfactory causal chain but in its pragmatic rationale. It has had to admit itself unable either to cure or to prevent the disease (2002: 4).

Traditional healers provide a unique opportunity for reaching rural populations that lie beyond the reach of urban-oriented public health services and national Information, Education and Communication (IEC) messages. Allen and Heald (2004: 1146) discuss the lack of AIDS awareness signs and postings in the rural part of Botswana. There is a coterie of traditional healers in every village; by tapping into this source of communication with the people, public health officials may well bridge the gap between evidence-based public health messages and the rural population in countries not altogether unlike Botswana.

Another explanation of Batswana choosing to access traditional healers services may be that they feel ill-at-ease or uncomfortable with allopathic doctors in urban clinics or hospitals. Rural Batswana consider urban hospitals to be, as one of our respondents put it, "places where one goes to die." Issues of language, communication, cultural codes, privacy, poor facilities, the desire for immediate relief, and belief in African explanations of illness are all reasons that patients may choose a traditional healer over a allopathic doctor (Fako, Linn & Brown 2000: 302 ff.). Not only is the traditional healer is able to explain the illness in terms that local culture can understand, but there is also the element of trust, as traditional healers often do not advertise but gain their clientele by word of mouth, therefore the healer has already been "vouched for" within the community.

Methods

Data for this chapter was collected from Mogoditshane, the largest peri-urban settlement outside Gaborone, the capital of Botswana. In 2006, the initial mapping process took place, which aimed at identifying traditional healers to be interviewed in the second stage of the study in 2008. This revealed that there were well over 100 traditional healers of various sorts; in the same geographic area, there were less than 10 allopathic clinics.

In mapping Mogoditshane, researchers entered the *location* as well as the *type of healer* and *basic contact information* into a "Google Earth" map; the mapping was preliminary and by no means exhaustive. Though useful for the next stage of research in 2008, this exercise suggested that traditional healing clinics were plentiful, diverse, often clustered (see Illustration 1), often more expensive than allopathic clinics, often operating in the evenings and sometimes well into the night and that many traditional healers have additional forms of employment.

Figure 5: Google Earth Map of Mogoditshane. Preliminary Mapping of Government Health Clinics (GOVT Clinic), Churches or Faith-based Organizations and Traditional Healers (TH).

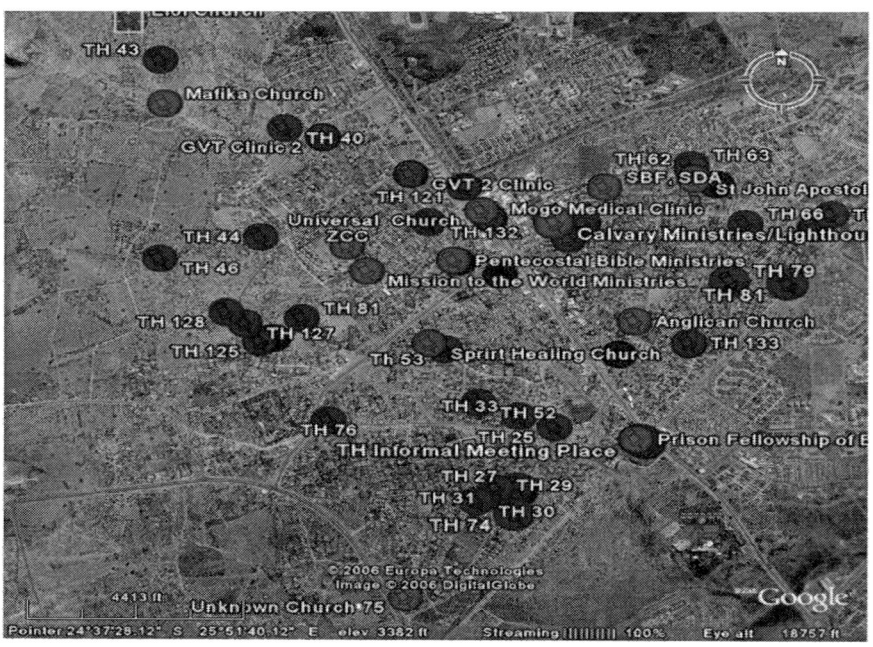

Thirty interviews were conducted with traditional healers, *Sangomas* and Prophets between January and March of 2008. The interviews with the traditional healers occurred at the locations where they provide their services. Traditional healers who had been practicing for longer periods of time, with a minimum of five years of practice, were sought out with the hope of gaining richer responses. Only a handful of younger healers, with less than five years of experience, were interviewed with the aim of gaining the ideas and attitudes of the next generation of healers.

Healers were identified primarily through the snowballing method and convenience sampling. With snowballing we were able to locate new healers through those already interviewed (Mack et al 2005: 5). Convenience sampling involved driving through the neighborhoods of Mogoditsane in a local style car and asking people (usually elders and often women) if they could direct us to a traditional healer in the neighborhood. A handful of these healers advertised on sign boards, which to other healers reflects poor skills, as it is believed that one should receive patients due to recommendations, not advertising.

The objective of the study was explained in Setswana or English and the traditional healers were given the option to participate in the study. Interviews began with close-ended questions intended to gather background information about the participant such as age, nationality, education, type of healer, etc. Then the interview moved into more opened ended questions focusing on the healer's practices and knowledge relating to HIV and AIDS and also experience and attitudes towards clinics and collaboration with allopathic doctors. The semi-structured questionnaire contained a set of open-ended questions designed to enhance the healer's freedom of expression and ailment conceptualization or etiology. The questionnaire was divided into five sections: demographic information, diagnostic and management practices, disease etiology, HIV and AIDS and collaboration. Some of the interview questions, slightly altered, were asked in more than one section of the questionnaire in order to gauge the consistency of the responses. The average interview, conducted either in Setswana or English, took about one hour. All of the interviews were audiotaped, transcribed and coded. The data collected was analyzed manually by the study team. The traditional healers were anonymous and therefore were assigned numbers 1-30. The reference TH 8, TH14, etc. refers to traditional healer number 8 or number 14, etc.

To augment the study findings, ten key informants who represent the formal health systems in Botswana were also interviewed using semi-structured questionnaires. The interviews with the key informants included Ministry of Health staff, UNDP staff in the HIV and AIDS unit, Western doctors working in the hospital closest to Mogoditsane, non-contract staff at the UN, the President of the Dingaka Tsa Setso association, staff from the Baylor Pediatrics Clinic, and an individual whose father was a traditional healer. Key informants were also located through the snowballing method. The purpose of these non formal semi-structured interviews was to gain insight into the local perceptions towards traditional healers at varying levels within the community. This exercise also provided a means to verify information from the secondary literature and to answer any questions that had risen from literature or previous interviews.

Study Findings

This section provides a selection of the preliminary results drawn from the primary data relevant to perceptions of HIV and AIDS (i.e., the etiology and origin of HIV, the effectiveness of anti-retroviral treatment and the limits of traditional medicine), present treatment practices, including referrals to allopathic clinics and psycho-social support, and the prospects – including inducements and obstacles – for collaboration between traditional and allopathic medical practitioners.

Desire to Further Understand AIDS

One of the initial items of the questionnaire asks directly "What is HIV/AIDS?" Among the 30 healers interviewed, one sixth of the respondents stated that they did not know what AIDS was, to which certain respondents added "only the whites know about it" (TH 3). Of those healers interviewed, 26% said that HIV could be transferred through cuts and wounds, 50% said that AIDS is a virus, and 86% of the healers said that the disease is sexually transmitted. 60% of the respondents identified condoms as an effective means of prevention and 23% discussed the need for a reduction in the number of sexual partners. Although most of the healers who were interviewed were familiar with the basic public health prevention messages about HIV, which they had heard over the radio or seen on a billboard, very few of the healers could provide a bio-medical description of HIV/AIDS. One healer commented that "AIDS has not been explained to the public in full detail, what it is, where it comes from and how it came about. When people started talking about it, he couldn't even understand what it was" (TH 1). Several respondents claimed that HIV was brought by the white people, others thought it was a mix of old diseases while some thought it was punishment for immoral behavior. Several of the healers discussed their disbelief when they first learned about AIDS through radio and media messages. It was only after they started seeing the sick people that they acknowledged the reality of the disease. Others discussed their bafflement concerning why some people caught the disease while others did not.

The majority of the healers suggested that traditional healers and traditional medicines cannot cure AIDS and, indeed, many warned that "any healer claiming to cure AIDS is lying." Only one of the respondents claimed that they could cure AIDS. On several occasions, the respondents expressed an interest in knowing why a cure had not yet been found for AIDS. They mentioned other diseases such as leprosy, malaria and Ebola, all of which had been problematic but manageable. They wanted to know why AIDS was giving them such a hard time.

Suspicion of the Origin of AIDS

Throughout the interviews the healers' suspicions about AIDS became evident. The area of greatest concern was the origin of the disease. Several of the healers expressed their suspicion that AIDS had come from condoms, birth control or pills administered from the hospital. TH 1 stated that he sometimes thinks that "AIDS may have come from all these tablets given at the hospital." This idea may well illustrate a deep-seated frustration toward allopathic practitioners for downplaying the role of traditional healers or, alternatively, express a lack of understanding of medicinal value of anti-retrovirals. One respondent commented: "This thing called AIDS, it never used to be there. You see, when they started bringing all the condoms, lubes, injections…you started hearing about AIDS" (TH 9). Other healers mentioned the fact that birth control and AIDS emerged at about the same time. Some healers said that regulating a woman's ability to get pregnant was "unnatural." Though it might be tempting to claim that these suspicions are the result of mistaking temporal associations or concurrence with causal explanation, we believe – with Ingstad (1989, 1990) – that these observations are insightful. Others expressed the belief that 'whites,' or medical doctors, may have more knowledge of the disease than what they are sharing. Healer 12 stated, "They don't want to tell us what AIDS really is." During the interviews some of the healers probed the researchers to see if we possessed any of this 'extra knowledge.' There seemed to be lingering suspicions concerning how it is that doctors can make a pill to control the symptoms associated with AIDS but cannot cure it.

Linking AIDS with Tswana Diseases

In an effort to understand HIV and AIDS, many of the traditional healers we interviewed linked AIDS with traditional or older Tswana diseases. The traditional healers were quick to identify "dirty blood" as the main factor responsible for transmission of AIDS. "AIDS is just contaminated blood" (TH 1). Dirty blood is representative of Tswana disease etiology; the health of an individual is centered on the blood (*madi*) which is seen as the life force (Haram 1991: 171). "Dirty blood coming into contact with a man, that is, *bolwetsi*, and then people call it AIDS even though there is no AIDS there" (TH 8). The transmission of HIV through intercourse is seen as a result of the blood mixing between the man and the woman, not as a result of infected semen or vaginal fluid. "Mostly, it (i.e., HIV) goes through the blood, so if you're circumcised the disease will still affect you" (TH 8).

Many of the healers thought AIDS was a mixture of diseases. "AIDS is a mixture of STDs inside a person's body which ends up being HIV/AIDS. Back then AIDS was not known to them just known to them as STDs such as gonorrhea, syphilis… Now there is no STDs, just AIDS; if you have sex with a person who is infected you just get AIDS" (TH 12). Traditional healers recognize some of the symptoms associated with AIDS to be similar to previous diseases, especially STDs, and suggest that AIDS is a combination of STDs. And indeed, biomedical researchers have similarly demonstrated an increased susceptibility to acquiring HIV if you have other STDs (see Shelton et al 2004: 891). The result of this belief, it seems, is that a few of the traditional healers thought AIDS was curable by attending to the elemental or pre-combinational ailments. "AIDS is curable because it's a combination of diseases. It's curable, you won't get cured right there, if you take your medication as told we will be fighting the diseases in the body step by step until it is just the virus alone…it doesn't just die there, it takes time to die" (TH 5).

Many of the respondents associated HIV and AIDS with *boswagadi*, a disease that occurs when a widow or widower does not undergo the treatment (i.e., the cleansing rituals) by which the "blood gets cleansed, (and by which) the man's blood comes out of the woman" (TH 13). There were varied explanations of how AIDS is tied to *boswagadi*: "AIDS is *bolwetsi*, it's *boswagadi*, it's when one dies and their partner is not treated, it's AIDS" (TH 7). "If somebody has not been treated for *boswagadi* and has sex, they can make another person sick with AIDS or other diseases" (TH 1). The belief that AIDS is *boswagadi* was more prominent among the older respondents.

Some healers attributed the arrival of AIDS to the morals adopted by the younger generations. "If this disease occurred longer ago it would have been a lesser problem because people had more control over their children and there would have been more successful attempts at encouraging abstinence through morals and values respected by the culture" (TH 1). Healer 15 stated, "You see, today's kids are very easy; you can get a girl very easy. Today's girls are very cheap; you see a girl getting very thin" (implying sick with AIDS).

Perception that Traditional Protection and Witchcraft does not apply to AIDS

Although most of the healers used traditional Tswana disease beliefs to explain the disease, many of them suggested that traditional "protection" remedies and witchcraft were ineffective when applied to AIDS. Many, if not most, of the healers we interviewed offered "protection" as one of their most valuable – and expensive – services. Protection is often used to guard cattle ranches, protect new businesses from thieves, protect against illness and some even use it to insure their cars against accidents. Healer 3 stated, "There is no way that we, as traditional healers, can protect against AIDS." Healer 8 warned that "A person who thinks that they are protected will go and have unprotected sex." There is a strong desire in Tswana culture to know the originating or ultimate cause of an ailment (see Livingston 2006: 78); often, the originating cause is identified with witchcraft (*boloi*). Many of the healers we interviewed, however, claimed that these traditional ideas do not apply to HIV and AIDS. "There is no AIDS because you have been bewitched…the only protection I can advise is the condom" (TH 12). This is an important concession, certainly, because it discourages the irresponsible sexual behavior that could result from a false sense of protection.

Perception that ARVs are Working

Most of the traditional healers we interviewed claimed that they cannot cure AIDS, which has led to a general acceptance of anti-retroviral drugs amongst traditional healers. "The best thing is to go to the clinic and get the pills. See if you can live longer, because you live up to 10 years with the virus" (TH 16). The healers recognized that these pills do not cure the disease but only increase the life span of the individual. "The Western doctors do not heal AIDS, all they do is make the symptoms go away" (TH 1). This recognition is important as it reinforces the magnitude of the disease and its incurability.

Treating HIV and AIDS patients

Many of the healers discussed ways in which they treat patients with AIDS. Often the healers discussed taking the traditional treatments in conjunction with ARVs. Healer 5 states, "It's okay to combine both medications, but you must follow the prescribed way of taking them." Healer 25 discussed treating patients with herbs to increase their appetite.

Some of the healers discussed doing physical therapy on patients on ARVs and using massage techniques to make them more comfortable. Several of the healers discussed traditional treatments that raised their patients' CD4 counts. Healer 21 discussed providing patients with medication that would treat other related diseases like diarrhea and STDs. According to Green, but based on his experience elsewhere (e.g., Uganda as well as Swaziland and Mozambique), most STD cases are taken to traditional healers, not to allopathic clinics (1994:2).

Referring Patients to the Clinic

The most common response encountered during the interviews when discussing how healers deal with AIDS patients was the referral of patients to clinics to learn their status and receive ARVs. Healer 17 commented that "For those with AIDS I don't waste their time, I tell them to go to the clinic." Healers were often sensitive about referring patients to the clinic. Most healers shared a reluctance to tell their patients that they suspected they were HIV positive; instead they would defer the responsibility of informing the patients of their status to the clinics. Healer 13 recounted how he "tells patients to go to the clinic in a very confidential way, he doesn't directly indicate that he suspects they have AIDS." Healer 17 commented that it is best to let the clinic tell them because patients may have "a short temper." Healer 13 suggested that the clinic was well equipped to deal with telling the patients; she had been there and felt "the counseling was so lively and cheerful ... they laugh, it's a good atmosphere."

The healers also play a role in recognizing when a patient may be infected and recommending they get tested so they can begin treatment as soon as possible. This is important as many of the healers discussed that they received patients who had not considered themselves at risk for being HIV positive but when the patient did not respond to the usual methods of healing, this often alerted the healers to the likelihood that it was the symptoms of AIDS they were dealing with.

Providing Spiritual Support and Counseling

One of the most significant roles of traditional healers in response to the HIV and AIDS crisis is the ability to provide counseling and spiritual support to those who may be too scared to test and for those who have already been diagnosed as HIV positive. Comments and conversations during interviews highlighted the deep fear amongst Batswana of contracting AIDS. Even the healers themselves expressed deep fear of AIDS. Healer 13 commented that "I fear this disease; I don't know where to run. The only way out for me is to be dead, and then it (AIDS) can never get me." Healer 3 commented that she will accompany patients to the clinic when they are too scared to go and test. This kind of personal support seems to be lacking at the clinic which is considered by many to be impersonal and staffed by inconsiderate health workers (Freeman and Motsei 1992: 1186). Healer 27 says that most of the AIDS patients are scared of the clinic. Healer 16 says that she will sit with them at the hospital, giving them love and motivation to stay strong. With the strong negative stereotypes that surround HIV and AIDS, this is an important role of providing support to those who are HIV positive. "If you give them (those already infected) spiritual love and patience it's even better than medication" (TH 13).

The healers also provide advice to patients, such as maintaining healthy diets, discussing their status with their partners, using condoms and continuing to take the ARVs. Healer 11 felt that "the role of traditional healers should be counseling. To advise people that they should not give up on life when they are taking these pills, to avoid stress, abstain from drugs and to eat healthier food with less sugar and oil." With the lack of staff and the aversion to clinics, healers play an important role in counseling HIV positive patients and encouraging healthy behavior. Botswana has a well developed ARV program to administer the drugs and provide counseling and testing centers. However, the program is a system designed for the masses. Traditional healers offer valuable services at an individual and community level.

Attitudes towards clinics and collaboration

Another part of the study focused on examining ideas and attitudes towards the Western allopathic clinics and the possibility of collaboration. In general, as discussed above, the traditional healers identified positive aspects of the clinics. The healers felt that clinics were able to handle illnesses that they themselves were not able to heal, but also felt that they were able to cure illnesses that clinics could not handle. They wished the clinic would recognize their ability to handle diseases that the clinic cannot treat. Healer 4 commented "It's possible that a traditional healer can be able to treat some diseases that Western doctors cannot treat." Healer 11 discussed a patient that "came to him with a natural disease, which the clinic called a migraine and gave her pills for 13 years...I treated her and now she doesn't take the pills no more, she was about to lose her sight." Healers stated that there were certain illnesses viewed to be Tswana diseases that foreigners could not handle, such as *sejeso* (food poisoning) or *ngoto* (constant nose bleed) or certain STDs which they could cure much more quickly.

Views of Western Medicine

One of the criticisms of Western medicine raised by the respondents was that it doesn't heal or cure illnesses, it just addresses the symptoms. Healer 8 commented that "Western clinic reduces the impact but does not heal or get rid of. See our way of operation, we heal permanently, but at the hospital, most of their herbs reduce the impact and then the pain comes back again and people sort of end up losing faith (in the clinic)." Perhaps this idea could be linked to arrival of ARVs and the healer's knowledge of ARVs inability to cure AIDS. Previous literature has discussed how patients may visit Western doctors to relieve symptoms but treatment by a traditional doctor is considered necessary to treat the real cause of the illness and bring a lasting cure (Steen and Mazonde 1999: 166). There has also been criticism of the medical doctors cutting out cancer instead of healing it and performing caesarian delivery instead of using massage to put the baby in the correct position. These lines of thought are more indicative of the healer's feeling that illness should be treated as a whole instead of just treating the symptoms.

Perceived Problems with the Clinics

The traditional healers were quick to point out the challenges of attaining health care at one of the hospitals or clinics. Most often the criticisms were about the inability to handle the sheer number of all of the patients. "Because all the clinics in Botswana are in short supply of doctors, sometimes when you go to the clinic, you find many patients and no doctor" (TH 4). Healers commented that there is a lack of doctors, extremely long lines, nurses doing work that a doctor should be handling and doctors being too slow and lazy. "Sometimes they are very slow at the hospital here. They should help them quicker...They take long" (TH 16). Another common complaint was the lack of individual attention from the doctor. "Western doctors don't attend to somebody individually. When you go to the clinic you may see 5 different people (helping you). When you go to a traditional healer, you get helped by one and it's not that you have to go looking for a doctor. If you come to my side, you come to my side alone" (TH 12).

Due to the challenges discussed and probably many other reasons, it appears that Batswana have developed a fear of going to the hospital or clinic and waiting until one is very ill. "Some are afraid of the clinic so they run to us" (TH 10). "People they just hide in their house and get eaten by the disease" (TH 19). Shame and stigma most likely play a strong role in people not wanting to acknowledge they have the virus.

Attitudes toward Collaboration

The majority of the healers expressed positive attitudes towards collaboration and working together to fight AIDS and other diseases. An interest and willingness of traditional healers to collaborate with allopathic doctors has been illustrated in many studies (Green and Makhubu 1984; Peltzer, Mnqqundaniso and Petros 2006; Rekdal 1999). Many of the healers welcomed collaboration and thought it was an excellent way to help their patients and improve their knowledge. One of the areas that healers expressed interest in was gaining more knowledge in measuring the amount of medicine to give to patients. "Yes I think it would be beneficial to us...because due to lack of education, we sometimes overdose prescriptions and I think the medical doctors can come in handy in this area to help us determine the dosage amount of our medications" (TH 8). Healers also discussed teaching the medical doctors about their medicine. "Western medicine has no clue, they cut out the disease (tumor), and we treat with herbs. But we could help teach them about the herbs. Herbs kill roots (the root of the disease). The medical doctors are very appreciative of this and they realize that this is very intelligent" (TH 8). Many showed interest in sharing knowledge. "It would make good sense to see more cooperation to check each other's progress being made. Now you cannot go to them, we die with our experience" (TH 14).

The healers expressed different interests in the role they would like to play in collaboration. Many talked about being able to send sick patients they could not cure to the hospital and to be called upon for patients that Western medicine was unable to cure. Healers talked about wishing to be able to carry their traditional herbs to the hospital and help patients there as well as receive them at home. Some healers talked about wanting to maintain a role as a social counselor. Most important to the healers was the ability to exchange knowledge freely. A majority of the healers stated that they wanted to meet with medical doctors and "sit down and talk." They want to share information about the illnesses they encounter and how to respond to them as well as teach the medical doctors how to address illnesses such as cancer from a more holistic perspective. They welcomed a forum in which they could talk. The majority felt that there is no opportunity to speak with medical doctors these days. Many healers felt that coming together would truly benefit the country. Collaboration could decrease the burden on the medical facilities, improve the medical conditions of patients, provide access to more holistic treatment and some traditional healers even claimed that they thought it could reduce government costs towards health care.

Challenges of Collaboration perceived by Traditional Healers

The traditional healers also identified possible complications of collaboration. The most challenging complication is that many healers felt that medical doctors did not consider their means of practice as a valid source of healing and many felt that the medical doctors had a condescending attitude. "We won't be taken as seriously as the medical doctors: if you look closely, the traditional healers are being looked down on and the clinics are not" (TH 5). The condescending attitude led many healers to feel discouraged at the idea of working together. "We don't have that cooperation with them because they think they are the ones who know all; they think they are the professors" (TH 7). Many healers discussed their frustration of referring their patients to the clinic to have a certain illness addressed, but the clinic never referring patients back to them. Healers also felt that medical doctors received more protection from the government than they did. "Take a situation where a healer treats a person and they die. When a medical doctor treats a person and they die, the community will not question the medical doctor" (TH 6). This idea was expressed many times. Most healers said their primary reason in joining the Traditional Healer Associations was to receive legal protection.

Healers of other nationalities that were residing and working in Botswana discussed how, in their countries, traditional healers were far more respected than in Botswana. A healer from Malawi discussed how hospitals and clinics in his country will call on traditional healers when they cannot solve certain health problems (TH 17). Healers from Zimbabwe pointed out that 'sick notes' from traditional healers were routinely accepted by Zimbabwean employers but not by Batswana employers.

Discussion

Ailments of various sorts are traditionally explicable as a consequence of disobeying or otherwise violating cultural taboos. The Mogoditshane

Study seems to confirm much of what has been observed by other researchers (e.g., Ingstad, 1990; Heald, 2000; Werbner, 1999; and Livingston, 2006). Ingstad's descripton, in 1990, of *meila* is still helpful:

> Concepts of disease transmission have mainly been connected with concepts of pollution that originate in the female body. This type of pollution may be transmitted to men via sexual intercourse that takes place within culturally proscribed periods after birth, abortion, etc. and before ritual purification has taken place. The man, through sexual intercourse, may then transmit the pollution to other women. Pollution that is caused by such violation of sexual taboos is called *meila*... Blood and semen are seen as the basic vehicles for transmission of the pollution (Ingstad 1990: 33).

These traditions limit and control sexuality. Each type of taboo violation is clearly defined with a Tswana name and in some cases specific types of symptoms. For example, when an individual is afflicted with *boswagadi,* her mere presence or proximity poses a threat to small children, livestock and crops. To overcome *boswagadi,* traditional healers prescribe one year of sexual abstinence in addition to certain purification rituals (Ingstad, Bruun and Tlou 1997: 366). It has been said that AIDS is *boswagadi* which has been brought about by the increasing number of young people becoming widows after drunk driving accidents and other ailments of modernization and not bothering to go through the proper period of sexual abstinence and purification rituals (Ingstad, Bruun and Tlou 1997: 365).

One of the challenges of the arrival of HIV and AIDS has been that the virus has many similarities with the Tswana diseases and has therefore caused confusion of whether HIV and AIDS is indeed a new disease or a culmination of the old Tswana diseases. And indeed, most of the respondents in Mogoditshane viewed AIDS as a variation on *boswagadi*. Rather than viewing this as 'an obstacle to collaboration,' one may well view it as an opportunity. As Ingstad observes:

> There is a striking similarity between ideas of disease transmission and *meila* in the Tswana medical system and notions of AIDS transmission in biomedicine. In both conceptual systems, sexual intercourse, blood and transmission from mothers to their babies play a role. Also in both systems disease and AIDS are strongly associated with violation of the sexual rules of society (1990: 34).

Traditional healers have tried to understand HIV and AIDS with its similarities to other sexual diseases and have sought to identify it with diseases they already know. Within the scientific framework there is a lack of satisfactory answers that make sense for people (Benn 2002: 9). One of the factors that make HIV and AIDS so difficult to explain is the factor of probability. Benn discusses an example of villagers knowing a certain woman is HIV positive, yet none of the men she has slept with have developed symptoms of the disease (2002: 10). This kind of non-consistency, an HIV positive woman not spreading the disease to men she has slept with, causes people and healers to link the illness with other factors such as breaking sexual taboos, witchcraft or another context in which they can explain the disease.

Although traditional healers may well lack a "comprehensive understanding of HIV and AIDS," at least from an allopathic if not also distinctively Western point of view, the study suggests that there is a sincere interest among Batswana *Dingaka ya Setso* in gaining more knowledge about the virus and collaborating with allopathic practitioners. Because traditional healers have access to a large proportion of the population, collaboration provides an excellent opportunity for reaching rural populations and sharing knowledge of AIDS and prevention practices. Unlike its neighboring countries, Botswana has been reluctant to engage in any collaborative efforts with traditional healers. Instead of trying to work with the traditional healers and improve their knowledge, the government has taken measures to control and regulate traditional healers in Botswana. In mid 2007, the Minister of Health, Professor Sheila Dinotshe Tlou, discussed her intentions to draft a law to regulate traditional medical practitioners (Lute 2007: 5). The government has stated that it believes "the two systems (traditional and modern medicine) cannot be integrated since they have different work ethics and belief systems. The present government policy is that the two systems should grow and develop separately" (Mafoko 2007: 5). The government explains its reluctance to engage with traditional healers: they cite their concern that traditional healers are – in some cases – taking financial advantage of their clients, that their practices may be unsafe and that they are not truly healers.

The Ministry cites concern for the wellbeing of its citizens from swindling doctors as the underlying cause for such regulation (Lute 2007: 5). Fees charged by traditional healer are relatively high, especially especially in contrast to the free medical care administered at hospital and clinics. However, this does not discourage the patients from seeking out traditional healers. In an interview at Princess Marina hospital in Gaborone, one of the doctors stated that patients often complain about having to pay the bus fare – which is equivalent to less than one US dollar – to go to the hospital, but yet they would save up and spend a considerable amount – often upward to fifty US dollars – to visit a traditional healer (Han 2008). If the government's main concern is people being financially taken advantage of, then collaboration would prove an excellent means to control such high fees. The hospital could recommend traditional healers who would be paid on a set fee scale and therefore would avoid the problem.

Another concern of the government is that traditional healing may be unsafe. It is true that research has proven that practices of traditional healers can make patients ill through practices such as sharing razor blades amongst patients, encouraging patients to take medicine which may make them sicker, prescribing dangerously incorrect dosages of herbal remedies and other practices (De Smet 1991: 48). This is a logical concern as there has been research discussing these dangers. But it is also important to point out that many of the healers interviewed were aware of these dangers such as sharing razor blades and insisted on using new razors or patients bringing their own razors.

Finally, the government is concerned that some healers are not truly healers but charlatans taking advantage of the Batswana people by using traditional beliefs and ideas to make a profit. There may be healers who are unethical or not practicing traditional healing methods while claiming they do, but that does not provide grounds to discount and discredit the entire profession based on the actions of a small percentage of the population. Kealotswe, (2009), argues that one problem faced by traditional healers in their healing methods is that they use old traditional methods based on beliefs which do not consider the fact that the anatomy of modern people has changed due to the different diets from those of the past. The body of a patient, which has a lot of chemicals, which were not there in the past cannot react positively to many traditional herbs and medicines. Many traditional healers stick to their traditional understanding of health and healing without putting into consideration that the modern body has changed. Failure to heal leads to the conclusion that some healers are charlatans, yet they really do their best from their own worldview. Every type of practice has its less-than-ethical members. Rather, this should encourage further investigation and certification of true traditional healers to protect the Batswana from engaging with the unscrupulous ones.

All of these points highlight the need for collaboration or, at the very least, more fruitful discussions about mutual suspicions. Concerning cost issues, collaboration and recommendation through the hospital would create set fees and avoid patients being charged unreasonably. Concerns about traditional healers' practices being unsafe can be addressed by educating them on unsafe practices and investing time to make their practices safe. The healers themselves have shown interest in learning more from the medical doctors, specifically in the area of dosage. Concerns about charlatan doctors can be addressed by having an intense certification program which requires traditional healers to undergo an exam. Clearly if the interest of the government is to protect the people it should rather be engaging in practices with traditional healers rather than turning a blind eye. Collaboration would help strengthen the services of traditional healers and provide a safe and protective environment for Batswana (as well as non-Batswana who are living in Botswana).

Perhaps a more challenging issue to address would be the negative associations of traditional healing being viewed as "backward" and "undeveloped." Several key informants acknowledged that there exists an unspoken (social bias) that traditional healers are "backward." With Botswana's constant quest to be modern and developed it is not surprising that it has labeled healers as "undeveloped" as traditional healers' treatments are not the way of the West. The key informants claimed that an "educated" person would not go to a traditional healer but rather to the hospital or clinic. However, multiple statements were made by traditional healers during the interviews that they receive clients from many different backgrounds, including government officials and nurses who advocate against their services. This may be a more challenging problem to address but it also further indicates the need for collaboration as people continue to see healers despite the negative associations.

Conclusion

Traditional healers often have high levels of credibility and respect among the population they serve and can therefore disseminate knowledge of HIV and AIDS into the community. Traditional healers have the potential to adapt their message to HIV and AIDS without discrediting their own beliefs and paradigms (Benn 2002: 16). In order to change existing discourse for sexual behavior it is necessary to find a way of changing the discourses from within the communities (Ntseane and Preece 2005: 349). Throughout Africa many or most STD cases are brought to traditional healers, therefore it makes sense to involve healers in referral, treatment and encouraging behavior change (Green 2000: 1). Stated differently, Benn suggests neglecting traditional healers and their explanations for the phenomena of HIV and AIDS would be both counter-productive and costly (Benn 2002: 17). This chapter provides the results of an exploratory study of the practices and attitudes of traditional healers in Mogoditshane, Botswana. Because of the nature of this study, as both exploratory and preliminary, it suffers from many limitations; the observations made and conclusions suggested are, therefore, tentative in character. That said, this study agrees with the UNAIDS recommendation generated by regional studies, namely, that "[i]t is only with renewed enthusiasm and enhanced capacity to generate widespead involvement of traditional healers in all aspects of the response to AIDS that we can curb the spread of HIV and its devastating effects on individuals, families and communities" (2006: 40). This study demonstrates the willingness of traditional healers to collaborate with medical providers, but also portrays the challenges with acceptability of such collaboration by the medical community and goverment. These differences will need to be addressed in order to achieve a harmonized, wholistic health system that incorporates the traditional healer and medical services that the Batswana population seeks.

Bibliography

Airhihenbuwa, C. *Health and Culture: beyond the Western paradigm*, London: Sage Publications, 1995..

—. "Culturally appropriate AIDS prevention in urban Africa: Implication for health education." *African Urban Quarterly*. Vol. 6:1, 1991. 57-59

Benn, C. "The influence of cultural and religious frameworks on the future course of the HIV/AIDS pandemic," *Journal of Theology for Southern Africa*, Vol. 113, 2002, 3-18.

Bulmer, M. and Warwick, D. (eds) *Social Research in Developing Countries: surveys and censuses in the third world,* London: Routledge, 1993.

Byaruhanga, A.B.T and Kealotswe, O. *African Theology of Healing*. Gaborone: Printworld, 1995.

Camaroff, J. *Body of Power, Spirit of Resistance*. Chicago: University of Chicago Press, 1985.

Chavunduka, G. *Traditional Medicine in Modern Zimbabwe,* Harare: University of Zimbabwe Publications, 1994.

De Smet, P. "Is there any danger in using traditional remedies?" *Journal of Ethnopharmacology*, Vol. 32, 1991. 43-50.

Fako, T., Linn, J., & Brown, B. "Transferring health technology to south Africa: the importance of traditional African culture," *Journal of Technology Transfer,* Vol. 25, 2000, 299-305.

Green, E.C. and Makhubu, L."Traditional healers in Swaziland: toward improved cooperation between the traditional and modern health sectors," *Social Science and Medicine*, Vol. 18:12, 1984, 1071-1079.

Green, E. *AIDS and STDs in Africa: bridging the gap between traditional healing and modern medicine,* Boulder: Westview Press, 1994.

—. *Indigenous Theories of Contagious Disease,* California: Alta Mira Press, 1999.

—. "Traditional Healers and AIDS in Uganda." *The Journal of Alternative and Complementary Medicine,* Vol. 6:1, 2000, 1-2.

Handwerker, W. Penn and Wozniak, Danielle "Sampling Strategies for the Collection of Cultural Data: An Extension of Boas's Answer to Galton's Problem," *Current Anthropology,* Vol. 38: 5, 1997, 869-875.

Ingstad B. "Healer, Witch, Prophet or Modern Health Worker? The Changing Role of *Ngaka ya* Setswana" in Jacobson-Widding, A. and Westerlund, D. (eds), *Culture, Experience and Pluralism: Essays on African Ideas of Illness and Healin.,* Stockholm: Almqvist & Wiksell International, 1989.

—. The Cultural Dimension of AIDS and its consequences for Prevention in Botswana. *Medical Anthropology Quarterly* 4:1, 1990, 28-40.

Ingstad, B. and Tlou, S. "AIDS and the elderly Tswana: The concept of pollution and consequences for AIDS prevention," *Journal of Cross-cultural Gerontology,* Vol. 12:4, 1997, 375-372.

Kealotswe, O. "Prophecy and Divination in New Religious Movements in Botswana: A Study of the similarities and differences between traditional healers and church prophets in Botswana," in *Aspects of New Religious Movements in Botswana,* Gaborone, Morula Series, Department of Theology and Religious Studies, University of Botswana, 2009 .

Kleinman, A., Einsenberg, L., "Good, B. Culture, Illness, and Care: Clinical Lessons from Anthropologic and Cross-Cultural Research," *Annals of Internal Medicine* Vol. 88, 1978, 251-258.

Last, M. "The Professionalization of African Medicine: Ambiguities and Definitions," in Last, M. and Chavunduka, G.L. (eds), *The Professionalization of African Medicine,* Manchester: Manchester Univ. Press, 1986, 1-19.

Livingston, J. *Morality and Debility in Botswana,* Indianapolis: Indiana Press, 2006.

Lute, A. "Traditional doctors to be regulated," Botswana Gazette ,Wednesday 06-12 June 2007, 5.

Mafoko, E. "Traditional Health Practitioners Seek Legislation," *Health News and Views* Vol. 17:1, 2007, 4-5.

Mikkelsen, B. *Methods for Development Work and Research: a new guide for practitioners,* London: Sage Publications, 2005.

Ministry of Health, *Code of Ethics for Traditional Healers.* Ministry of Health, Gaborone, Botswana, 2004.

Neumann, A.K. and Lauro, P. "Ethnomedicine and Biomedicine Linking," *Social Science and Medicine* Vol. 16, 1982, 1817-1824.

Ntseane, P. and Preece, J. "Why HIV/AIDS prevention strategies fail in Botswana: considering discourses of sexuality," *Development Southern Africa*, Vol. 22:3, 2005, 347-363.

Nutbeam, D. and Harris, E. *Theory in a Nutshell: a practical guide to health promotion theories,* New York: McGraw Hill, 2004.

Peltzer, K., Mnqundaniso, N. and Petros, G. "HIV/ AIDS /TB knowledge, beliefs and practices of traditional healers in KwaZulu-Natal, South Africa," *AIDS Care* Vol. 18:6, 2006, 608-613.

Ragin, C. *Constructing Social Research*, London Pine: Forge Press, 1994.

Rekdal, O.B. "Cross-cultural healing in east Africa ethnography," *Medical Anthropology* Vol. 13, 1999, 458–461.

Republic of Botswana *Botswana AIDS Impact Survey II: Popular Report (BAIS II).* Republic of Botswana, Gaborone, Botswana, 2005.

Scheyvens, R. and Leslie, H. "Gender, Ethics and Empowerment: Dilemmas of Development Fieldwork," *Women's Studies International Forum* Vol. 23:1, 2000, 119-130.

Werbner, R. *Postcolonial Subjectivities in Africa*, London: ZED Books, 1999.

UNAIDS, *Ancient Remedies, New Disease: Involving traditional healers in increasing access to AIDS care and prevention in East Africa*, Geneva: UNAIDS, 2002.

—. Collaborating with Traditional Healers for HIV Prevention and Care in sub-Saharan Africa, http://data.unaids.org/Publications/IRC-pub01/JC299-TradHeal_en.pdf, 2006.

WHO. *Traditional Medicine Programme & Global Programme on AIDS: Report of the Consultation of AIDS and Traditional Medicine: prospects for involving traditional health practitioners*, Francistown: WHO, 1990.

WHO. *WHO Traditional Medicine Strategy 2002-2005*, Geneva: WHO, 2002.

CHAPTER TEN

FAITH BASED ORGANIZATIONS' APPROACHES IN THE FIGHT AGAINST HIV AND AIDS IN BOTSWANA: 1985-2009

JAMES NATHANIEL AMANZE

Introduction

Botswana will go down in history as one of the countries in the world, which had one of the highest prevalence rates of HIV and AIDS in proportion to its population. This chapter discusses the various strategies that Faith Based Organizations (FBOs) have adopted in the fight against the pandemic. It will be argued in this chapter that the Christian churches' understanding of the nature of human sexuality has limited, to a certain extent, their choices of the means and ways of combating the scourge. On the basis of some ethical considerations, they have resisted, for a very long time, the use of condoms as a preventative method against HIV and AIDS. However, because of the severity of the epidemic in the country, they opted to this measure as a matter of last resort. Some of the strategies in the fight against the HIV and AIDS scourge, which shall be discussed in this chapter, will include, among others, prayer, counseling, the establishment of day care centers, hospices, education of the masses by means of workshops, seminars and conferences and insistence on abstinence and behavior change in general. All in all, it will be shown in this chapter that FBOs have indeed a major role to play in the prevention, care, and treatment of people living with HIV and AIDS in Botswana today.

Human sexuality in the era of HIV and AIDS:
Voices from the churches

The HIV and AIDS pandemic in Botswana can be described as a national nightmare in the sense that it has affected the welfare of the whole country, socially, economically, politically, culturally and religiously. Although scientific factors that account to the emergence and spread of HIV and AIDS are common knowledge and though the nature of the epidemic, the fact that there is no cure for HIV and AIDS, and its methods of prevention are also in the public domain, the pandemic continues to spread at an alarming rate making Botswana one of the hardest hit countries in the world! As Oscar Motsumi once said "This country has been bombarded with HIV messages, but there hasn't been a change in behaviour" (http://www.avert.org/aidsbotswana.htm).

The fact that the HIV and AIDS pandemic spreads mainly through sexual intercourse, between a man and a woman (heterosexually) and between a man and another man (homosexually) victims of the epidemic were automatically stigmatized from the very beginning by the churches as well as the general public. The implication has been that the victims have been involved either in adulterous relationships, premarital sexual relationships or homosexual relationships. It is important to point out that one of the elements that determined the position of the churches in Botswana in regard to their response to the HIV and AIDS pandemic is their theology of human sexuality. The New Penguin English Dictionary (2000: 1282) has defined sexuality as the condition of having a sexual nature and experiencing sexual desires". It also means "a person's sexual orientation, as a heterosexual or a homosexual or sexual preferences". To a large extent, the churches' understanding of human sexuality has compelled them to reject methods of prevention, which appear contrary to the will of God. It is important here to reflect on the theology of human sexuality as expressed in different churches operating in Botswana today. The best way of doing this is to hear their voices concerning their understanding of human sexuality and its role in society.

In the first instance, the position of the Roman Catholic Church worldwide is that sex is a sacred gift from God and that it is entirely for procreation. Each sexual act must lead to the procreation of a human being in which case pre-marital and extra-marital sex is not allowed. In this regard, the Roman Catholic Church forbids its members from using contraceptives of any kind for any purpose whether within marriage or outside marriage. This is clearly stated in Pope Paul VI's Encyclical letter of regulations of births entitled *Humanae Vitae,* which was issued on 25th July 1968 concerning procreation and contraceptives according to which:

> .....commitment to responsible parenthood requires that husband and wife, ... Recognise their own duties towards God, themselves, their families and human society. From this it follows that they are not free to do as they like in the service of transmitting life, on the supposition that it is lawful for them to decide independently of other considerations what is the right course to follow. On the contrary, they are bound to ensure that what they do corresponds to the will of God the Creator....the Church in urging men to the observance of the precepts of the natural law teaches as absolutely required that in any use whatever of marriage there must be no impairment of its natural capacity to procreate human life (Flannery 1982:402).

On the basis of the theological position stated above, the Roman Catholic Church teaches its members to practice sacred sex and not safe sex. By safe sex the church understands sexual intercourse in which a person uses contraceptives in order to avoid either pregnancy or infection with sexually transmitted diseases such as HIV. The church considers this unacceptable because it impairs the natural capacity to procreate human life. Generally speaking, the church encourages sacred sex in the context of marriage because the Christian is the Body of Christ, the temple of the Holy Spirit (1 Cor. 7: 13-20); therefore, the body must be honoured and respected. The church is aware that we live today in an imperfect society. The society, which we live in is in a state of moral degradation. Sexual instincts are stimulated early in life as a result of peer pressure and other complex factors. However, the church insists that the faithful must do all they can not to engage in sexual immorality of any kind and live in accordance with God's will. This position is absolute whether one is living in the era of the HIV and AIDS pandemic or not (Corrigan, Interview).

This view of human sexuality is shared by other churches in Botswana though in slightly different ways. For example, the Anglican Church, which is traditionally known as the *Via Media* (The Middle Way) tries as much as possible to avoid the extremes of Roman Catholicism on the one hand and of Protestantism on the other. To this end, the Anglican Church's philosophy in dealing with issues that affect human sexuality especially in the era of HIV and AIDS pandemic is based on Thomas A Kempis thesis *The imitation of Christ* in which he noted that when we are faced with two evils we should always choose the less. As regards human sexuality, the Anglican Church teaches that sex is a sacred gift from God and that it must ideally only take place in marriage. Therefore, pre-marital and extra-marital sexual relationships are condemned as evil because they are contrary to the will of God in accordance with the teaching of the Bible. Having said this, however, the church is aware that sex is something that is always in the mind of the people. In this regard, the church holds the view that people have different inherent weaknesses one of which is the abuse and misuse of sex. The church is also aware that when people commit fornication and adultery they feel that they have done something wrong. The implication of this is that Batswana are aware that fornication and adultery are sinful. However, the church is aware that when people are engaged in pre-marital and extra-marital sex they are at the moment of their lowest weakness. In this regard, the church notes with concern that when it comes to matters of human sexuality, there are certain categories of people in society who are vulnerable. The powerful and the rich quite often, sexually abuse women, the poor, the powerless, and the marginalised. Therefore, they need protection from sexual abuses. Until the conditions that lead to unhealthy sexual relations are removed from our society, many people in Botswana will be exposed to the dangers of HIV and AIDS pandemic. The Anglican Church, therefore, does not condemn the use of contraceptives as a means of birth control either by married couples or single mothers. The church prefers the use of contraceptives as a mechanism of birth control rather than abortion, which is considered as infanticide. This approach is based on the church's awareness that we are not a perfect society. It is, therefore, necessary to concentrate on the less of two evils that will promote the "greater good". The greater good encapsulates all that God stands for, that is, grace, love, generosity, forgiveness and acceptance (Makhulu, Interview).

The sanctity of human sexuality and its unique position in the life of human societies has also been echoed in the United Congregational Church of Southern Africa (UCCSA). According to Rev. Rupert Hambira (Interview), one of the ministers of the UCCSA in Gaborone, the church teaches that sex is a gift from God and that it should not be used in a way that is contrary to the will of God. While it is understood that human sexuality is primarily for procreation, there is no official position in the United Congregational Church in Southern Africa regarding the use of contraceptives by Christians either for family planning or in order to protect them from the HIV and AIDS pandemic. This is because the UCCSA is founded on the principles of congregationalism according to which each congregation is independent in the sense that each body of worshippers or congregation is locally governed and only answerable to itself. The church teaches that Christians must abstain and be faithful to their partners. But the church is also aware that despite the good will and efforts of Christians to abstain from pre-marital and extra-marital sex, people are still engaging in illicit sex and in the process continue to be vulnerable to sexually transmitted diseases including HIV and AIDS. In recent times there has been a general understanding in the church that those who fail to abstain and to be faithful to one partner must of necessity use contraceptives in order to save their own lives and the lives of others.

According to Hambira, unless the conditions that lead to sexual abuse such as poverty, incest, rape, peer pressure, urbanisation, economic inequalities and corruptible programmes on TVs are removed, human sexuality will continue to be a source of misfortune and death. Hambira has observed that the Church must develop a theology of abstinence and faithfulness that can be applied not only to sexual matters but also to all other areas of human life. There must be faithfulness in all-human relationships. These morals, namely abstinence and faithfulness, must permeate all other human institutions. There must be alternatives in our society that can help young people to be away from conditions that lead them to sexual promiscuity. Abstinence is an end product of socialisation. Rev. Hambira pointed out to me that there are no structures in Botswana at present that can support the kind of life advocated in the church. The Church must lay a philosophical framework that can begin to influence and impact the way in which people live today without using the words abstinence and be faithful. Batswana need a philosophy to live by that can enhance the value of life for its own sake as a gift from God.

A similar view in regard to matters of human sexuality in church and society was expressed to me by Rev. O. E. Mere of the Methodist Church (Interview). According to Mere, the position of the Methodist Church in Southern Africa, which includes Botswana, looks at the question of human sexuality from different angles. Sex is a divine gift to humanity, which needs to be practiced responsibly. When it comes to the question of the use of contraceptives, the church looks at it from a situational ethical perspective. The question raised is "what is the current situation?" This is the bottom line of the matter. The focus is on the following three points. The first point consists of the biblical view of sex before marriage. In this regard, the church teaches that biblically unmarried people should abstain completely. But the prevailing situation in Botswana is that people are exposed to pornographic material on TV and other media. To counteract this state of affairs the church holds that as the TV people have commercialised pornography and other sexual materials; the church too should commercialise its teaching on sexual morality. The second point consists of sex within marriage. In this context the church holds that sex outside marriage is condemned on the basis of 2 Sam 11: 11 where Yahweh condemned David because of his adulterous relationship with

Bathsheba, Uriah's wife. The church emphasises that one should be faithful and stick to one partner. The third point consists of marriage in the African context where in some societies it is socially and legally allowed for a man to have multiple wives. The position of the church is that in an African context where polygamy is legally and socially sanctioned, the polygamist must be faithful to all his wives. In short, the church is not concerned with the number of wives a person has but the faithfulness and commitment to one another. The church emphasises faithfulness and fairness to the partners in a marriage context whether monogamous or polygamous. The church places emphasis on teaching and educating people on good moral sexual behaviour.

In the same vein, when it comes to matters of human sexuality, the Evangelical Lutheran Church in Southern Africa and in Botswana emphasises on the sacred nature of human sexuality and that its fulfillment should only occur in the context of marriage. Bishop Ntuping of the Evangelical Lutheran Church in Southern Africa, at one of the interviews I had with him, put it this way:

> We maintain that sex should happen in the context of marriage. So we are against sex outside marriage. On matters of sex, the Lutheran Church teaches people to exercise self-control. By this we mean that people who are not married should control their sexual behaviour. They should not be engaged in pre-marital sex but should wait until they get married. A person cannot die if he/she does not have sex. We teach our members that one man must have one wife and one woman must have one husband (Interview).

This view was echoed by Bishop John Robinson of the Lutheran Evangelical Church in Botswana according to whom the church takes into account seriously the fact that it deals with "fallen humanity", which is totally corrupt (Interview). According to Robinson, human beings are sinful for as long as they remain in this world. The position of the church on matters of human sexuality is based on Pauline theology. Paul writing to his followers in Corinth noted "I wish that all were as myself am. But each has his own special gift from God, one of one kind and one of another. To the unmarried and the widows I say that it is well for them to remain single as I do. But if they cannot exercise self-control, they should marry. For it is better to marry than to be aflame with passion (1 Cor. 7: 7-9)." In this context, the church holds the view that sexual desire must only be fulfilled in the context of marriage although the Church is aware that there are those who struggle in the path of Christ in which case the use of condoms may be required to prevent sexually transmitted diseases such as

HIV and AIDS. Bishop Robinson pointed out to me that the Church is of the view that unmarried couples must be guided together with the view towards getting married. This is what the church would prefer ultimately. This is the ideal situation.

The view concerning the special place of human sexuality in the divine scheme of creation was reiterated by Rev. Cloete of the Dutch Reformed Church according to whom when it comes to sexual matters, the church advises and encourages its unmarried members to abstain completely until marriage. This is because sex must only be practiced in the context of marriage (Interview). The church advises its unmarried members to seek for themselves suitable marriage partners who would also abstain because this is what God wills. The church wants its people to live the life of purity in accordance with the will of God. The church tries to help young people to develop health relationships with members of the opposite sex. Young people are encouraged to develop normal relationships in the pattern of the life of Jesus. They must court in the Christian way in preparation for their marriage. The church leadership, however, admits that despite this teaching young boys go on to make young girls pregnant.

Similarly, the Apostolic Faith Mission (AFM) teaches that sex outside marriage is immoral and unacceptable. Pastor Johannes Kwarapi, the Superintendent of the AFM, pointed out to me that the church emphasises that a Christian must be born again (Interview). The church of the born again Christians does not practice sex outside marriage. He further observed that the enemy number one of Botswana society is sin as seen in sex outside marriage. According to Kwarapi, the Bible teaches that the wages of sin is death; therefore, everybody who indulges himself/herself in sexual sin should know that the end result is death. People should know that the best way to avoid sexually transmitted diseases is God's way which is to abstain from sex (unmarried people) and be faithful to one's partner (married people).

This point has also been emphasised by members of the Assemblies of God Church in Botswana (Habibo, Interview). The church's position is that unmarried Christians must abstain from pre-marital sex and those who are married must always be faithful to their partners. This is because both pre-marital and extra-marital sexual relationships are considered immoral on the basis of the teaching of the Bible. Having said this, however, the church takes cognisance of the fact that human beings live in a fallen environment under the throes of Satan. This is evidenced by the fact that though the church preaches abstinence and faithfulness to one's wife or husband few people take this teaching seriously. People have rendered a deaf ear to the ethical teachings of the church.

Another church that stresses the sinful nature of pre-marital and extra-marital sexual relationships is the Seventh Day Adventist. According to the official position of this church world-wide, unmarried people should abstain from sex completely. It is argued that this is a philosophy that finds its roots in the Bible. It is also in harmony with God's will. The church teaches that sex should only be practiced among married people. Sex outside marriage is at odds with God's revealed purpose to human beings. As regards the use of contraceptives, the church leadership makes a subtle distinction between what is known as "the church position" and "individual practice". The church does not go on legislating individual or private behaviour. However, it is the church position that unmarried Christians should abstain from sex and those who are married must stick to their partners. This position is taken on the understanding that God never justifies human shortcomings in relation to his standing orders on moral issues. According to Pastor A. Mpofu (Interview), when God said, "you should not steal" there was no provision made that in certain circumstances a person can still because he/she is hungry. Everyone must abide by the standards set by God. Pastor Mpofu pointed out to me that the church teaches that people should abstain and be faithful to one's partner on the understanding that God himself will give them the grace and the strength to abstain. It is believed that with the power of prayer all things are possible with God. Pastor Mpofu, however, admitted that though the Church teaches that people should abstain nothing has been put in place to enable people to get away from sex and live up the standards set by the church.

This discussion would be incomplete without reflecting the views from one of the African Independent Churches in Botswana namely, St. Michael's Apostolic Church. According to Bishop Peterson Bothongo (Interview), the prevailing view in the African Independent Churches is that people should first marry and after marriage can have sex within marriage otherwise pre-marital and extra-marital sexual relationships would compromise Christian ethics. It is perceived in African Independent Churches that sexual immorality brings condemnation and judgment from God as witnessed with the advent of the HIV and AIDS pandemic. Judgment of their souls will come soon or later. It is argued that on matters of human sexuality, God's stand cannot be compromised as a result of present circumstances. St. Michael's Apostolic Church teaches that those who are not married must abstain completely from sex until marriage and those who are married must fulfill their sexual desires in marriage. This, of course, has its own implications. Bishop Bothongo is of the view that Christians must be counselled that when they embrace Jesus Christ as their personal Saviour, they must be prepared to make some sacrifices such as abstinence.

Christian views of human sexuality:
A pathway to stigma and discrimination

It will be seen from the above discussion that Faith Based Organizations in Botswana all agree in one thing, that sex is a gift from God and that pre-marital and extra-marital sex as well as homosexuality are unacceptable because they are contrary to the will of God. Although the interviews discussed above were conducted a decade ago, FBOs in Botswana have not changed in terms of their attitude to abstinence and faithfulness in marriage as the two preferred HIV prevention methods. In a more recent study Togarasei et al (2008) had similar findings. It follows then that the link between the HIV and AIDS on the one hand and sexual activity on the other has made FBOs consider the HIV and AIDS pandemic a disease of sinners and not a natural disease like any other in the world. Those who are infected, therefore, are generally perceived as living under divine retribution. This naturally leads to stigma and discrimination.

In the *Christian Ethics and HIV/AIDS* Amanze (2007:28-47) has argued that stigma is the greatest obstacle in the fight against the HIV and AIDS pandemic in Africa. The Christian view that human sexuality is a sacred gift from God and that sex can only be practiced in the context of marriage, authenticated the view that people living with HIV and AIDS broke the seventh commandment "Thou shall not commit adultery" and injunctions against fornication. The connection between sex and HIV and AIDS meant that those infected with HIV were considered as immoral at the highest degree. As a result, the initial attitude of Faith Based organizations in Botswana towards victims of HIV and AIDS was thoroughly negative. Since HIV and AIDS pandemic is transmitted primarily through sexual contact, PLWHA are generally perceived as the most sinful of all. Their illness and death are conceived as punishment from God the Master Creator. In other words, such people are said to have broken God's sacred laws of abstinence and sticking to one's wife or husband. This view has stigmatised many PLWHA to the extent that many of them have been driven underground. The stigma is of such proportion that when people, who have lost their beloved ones, are told that their relatives died from AIDS they refuse to accept the verdict. HIV and AIDS therefore has become a secret disease in which victims suffer and die with a sense of rejection by their own people among whom they were born, grew and lived. At the initial stages of the epidemic, Christian churches used to treat victims of HIV and AIDS with great disdain under the assumption that they committed a mortal sin, the sin of sexual immorality that sometimes is believed to have led to the fall of humanity in the Garden of Eden (Gen. 1: 1-7).

The responses of the churches, therefore, left much to be desired. It has been observed, for example, that in the era of HIV and AIDS, FBOs have not been very helpful in a number of ways. They have been accused of being a 'sleeping giant'; of promoting stigma and discrimination based on fear and prejudice; of promoting harsh moral judgments on those infected and affected; of obstructing the efforts of the secular world in the area of prevention especially in connection with the use of condoms and of reducing the issues of HIV and AIDS to simplistic moral pronouncements. These negative attitudes have made churches and mosques not places of refuge and solace but exclusion zones for the victims of the epidemic. The general conclusion has been that people living with HIV and AIDS are reaping the fruits of their sinful life especially their sexual immorality (Parry 2003). The slow reaction of the churches to tackle the problems stemming from the HIV and AIDS in Africa generally and Botswana in particular prompted the Executive Committee of the World Council of Churches to issue a warning as early as 1986 in the following words:

> Churches as institutions have been slow to speak and to act, that many Christians have been quick to judge and condemn many of the people who have fallen prey to the disease; and that through their silence, many churches share responsibility for the fear that has swept our world more quickly than the virus itself (WCC 2006:1).

With this concern in mind and with a spirit of great urgency, the WCC urged the churches in 1996 to promote both in their own lives and in the wider society, a climate of sensitive, factual and open exploration of the ethical issues posed by the pandemic and, in view of the prevailing stigma, encouraged the churches to formulate and advocate a clear policy of non-discrimination against people living with HIV and AIDS (WCC 2006:1). In this regard, the WCC's involvement in the fight against stigma and discrimination as well as its urge in formulating policies that promote prevention of the spread of HIV, mobilising of resources, advocating universal access to treatment has been total and felt everywhere. For example, in 2001 the General Secretary of the World Council of Churches, Dr. Konrad Raiser, joined hands with the Botswana Council of Churches (BCC) in its efforts to fight against the pandemic under the theme "Peace Making and Pastoral Care to Victims of Violence and HIV/AIDS". The program was intended to alleviate the untold suffering of the affected and infected and enable them to live positively.

Judgment gives way to compassion; condemnation to forgiveness

The magnitude of HIV and AIDS in Africa generally and Botswana in particular compelled Faith Based Organisations to take action against the epidemic. As it has been noted above, FBOs' theological stance on human sexuality generated a number of accusations against them. Having said this, however, it has also been noted that FBOs have done and are doing tremendous work to alleviate the suffering of those who are infected and affected by the HIV and AIDS pandemic. It has been observed that congregations and parishes have been in the front line of care and support right across Africa, of people living with HIV and AIDS. This is evidenced by the fact that a number of initiatives have been taken by the churches to fight against the epidemic (Parry 2003:3).

What has been said of Africa generally is true of Botswana, which has registered the highest number of HIV and AIDS prevalence rates in the world. It has been noted, however, that in the context of Botswana, with the government providing almost everything, it took a long time for the churches to take up the challenges of the epidemic. It took time for the churches to form collaborative efforts between the denominations to fill the gaps to supplement and complement the government efforts. The only good thing is that once they did so they managed to establish counseling services and networking that is second to none and has become a regional initiative stretching up to Liberia (Parry 2003:3).

Faith Based Organizations' responses to the HIV and AIDS pandemic in Botswana

Faith Based Organizations have adopted different strategies in the fight against HIV and AIDS. These include, prayer, education of the masses on HIV and AIDS issues through workshops and seminars, the establishment of day care centres for orphans, hospices, insistence on behavior change, provision of counseling services, conferences, youth initiatives, and in special circumstances the need to use condoms as when a partner (husband or wife) is HIV positive. We shall turn our attention to look at some of these.

Prayer as a means of fighting against HIV and AIDS

Prayer has been one of the most effective means in the fight against HIV and AIDS in Botswana. Batswana, being by nature religious, believe strongly in the power of prayer. In this regard, apart from the efforts made by the government to arrest and eventually eradicate HIV and AIDS, FBOs have also joined the fight by using spiritual means of combat. Once the ferocity of the epidemic became obvious, the churches in Botswana in consultation with government initiated annual prayers for the whole nation. September was designated as the month of prayer for HIV and AIDS victims. During the month of September FOBs intensify their campaign against HIV and AIDS. This is done through preaching, workshops, seminars and counseling in schools, prisons, hospitals, clinics, colleges and other public places. Prayers are organized every morning before commencing work in order to raise peoples' awareness of the dangers posed by the epidemic. People are encouraged to change their behavior especially on matters of human sexuality. Great emphasis is placed on abstinence and faithfulness to one partner over the use of condoms (Nkomazana 2007:56).

The education of the masses through workshops and seminars

One way in which FBOs in Botswana began to fight against HIV and AIDS was through education of the masses. This was done ecumenically through the Association of Medical Missions in Botswana. This association consists of several medical hospitals namely the Scottish Livingstone Hospital, Bamalete Lutheran Hospital, Debora Retief Memorial Hospital, St. Joseph's Mission Clinic, Seventh Day Adventist Hospital, Mission Dental Service, Botswana Adventist Medical Services, Flying Mission, Society for the Deaf, St. Conrad's Mission Clinic and Thuso Rehabilitation Centre. Having started as a wing of the Botswana Council of Churches, in the early 1970s the association acquired independent status and became a fully-fledged association. With the arrival of the HIV and AIDS pandemic in the country in the middle of 1980s the association turned its attention almost immediately to fight against the epidemic with all the available resources at its disposal. An AIDS working party was formed whose task was to educate people about HIV and AIDS and its prevention. As a matter of fact, as time went by this became one of the first priorities of the association. The AIDS working party conducted workshops, produced pamphlets, videos, badges, poetry and other means of communication about AIDS. In order to accomplish its works of mercy and compassion, the association received financial assistance from the Interchurch Organization for Development Cooperation (ICCO), MEDICUS MUNDI (both from the Netherlands) and the Norwegian Development Agency (NORAD) from Norway but based in Botswana (Amanze 1994:22-23). The Botswana Council of Churches through its different agencies and affiliates has insisted on the need for health education, general information campaigns, target group programmes with special work with workers in the private sector, peer education for youth and women, curriculum in secondary schools, training of teachers, out of school youth, traditional healers, commercial sex workers and truck drivers.

Insistence on behavior change

Since the beginning of the campaign, FBOs in Botswana have insisted that the first and major step to be taken in the fight against HIV and AIDS is behaviour change. Assembly after Assembly the Botswana Council of Churches has spoken, prophetically, against promiscuity and has urged Christians and the general public to change their sexual behaviour as the best way of fighting against the HIV and AIDS epidemic. Abstinence and the need to be faithful to one's partner have also been emphasised. This has been the primary message of the churches. With youth the strategy is to help them postpone their sexual activity until they get married. It is also felt that there is a need to encourage women to demand a change in sex-life inside marriage and to encourage people to change social norms, which accept many casual sexual partners. Prevention, sex education, as well as counselling for PLWHA and their families are felt essential. In this struggle against HIV and AIDS, the BCC has, quite often, assumed a co-ordinating role of the activities of the churches and serves as a major link with government (BCC 1993:3).

Adolescence Sexual Reproductive Health (ASRH)

Another response in the fight against HIV and AIDS has targeted young people through the Adolescence Sexual Reproductive Health (ASRH) program. The program was designed primarily for adolescents because of the various health problems that they face every day. The aims of the program are (a) to reach to in and out of school adolescents; (b) to educate them on growth and development, sexuality, sexually transmitted infections and HIV and AIDS prevention; (c) to give them skills for managing their own sexual lives including decision making, attitudes, values and behaviour on matters pertaining to alcohol, substance abuse, smoking and teenage pregnancies; and (d) to increase the use of sexual and reproductive health information and services. This program was established on the theological premise that God created people as sexual beings in his image and likeness (Gen. 1: 27-28) and that their sexuality is an integral part of their being. It is believed, therefore, that talking about human sexuality is not sinful and that it will help adolescents inside and outside the church to confront the challenges of life as adolescents. ASRH targets youth aged between 10 to 35 years. The aim is to help people to be very sensitive in approaching the youth so that they can speak to them in a language that is not insulting, does not stigmatise and does not alienate them. This approach, it is hoped, will help young people to change their sexual behaviour and stay alive (Modiega, Interview and Mokaedi).

In order to disseminate information to the youth a variety of venues are used which include homes, Sunday Schools, youth meetings, baptism, confirmation and catechetical classes, women's fellowship meetings, deacons meetings, church meetings, offices, schools, *kgotla* and other venues. In this program parents are urged to establish good communication with their children. They are urged to provide a friendly environment in their relationship with them so that they may open up and be able to discuss with them matters pertaining to human sexuality. It is argued that talking to children about sexuality does not encourage them to engage in sexual activities; rather it helps them to appreciate their own bodies and equips them with the knowledge and skills to say no to sex and not to be tricked into early sexual activity (ASRH, no date).

In order to carry out this program effectively, the UNFPA has, from time to time, made some donations to the BCC in an effort to assist the institution to work with adolescents and to create an enabling environment for promotion of sexual productive health. The money donated to the BCC assists the Council in the mainstreaming of broader Adolescent Sexual Reproductive Health issues into the activities of the Church. The task of the BCC in this partnership is to mobilise parents and the community in an effort to support ASHR initiatives. Additionally, the BCC is expected to develop membership policy guidelines on the mainstreaming and institutionalisation of ASHR programmes as well as creating a conducive environment for ASRH activities (Modiega, Interview).

Counseling people living with HIV and AIDS:
The role of BOCAIP

One of the FBOs, which has contributed substantially in the struggle
against HIV and AIDS, is the Botswana Christian AIDS Intervention
Program (BOCAIP). This is a Christian movement against AIDS in
Botswana. It operates in the form of a network. It is composed of local
Christian AIDS initiatives from across the country and other Christian
organizations and institutions. It also draws Christian individual
membership from varied sectors ranging from the university, private sector
and government. BOCAIP was founded in 1996 and was officially
registered in 1999. It is a non-governmental organization registered under
the Societies Act. The national coordination office works with nine
counseling centres in Maun, Molepolole, Ramotswa, Lobatse, Kanye,
Gaborone, Francistown, Masunga and Selebi-Phikwe. This FBO continues
to mobilize the rest of the country for the development of sustainable
community owned initiatives in other areas of Botswana. BOCAIP trains
counselors in HIV and AIDS issues from a Christian perspective. The
basic HIV and AIDS curriculum training manual of the Ministry of Health
as well as promotion of nutrition and health is used. Apart from this,
BOCAIP monitors and evaluates the centres. At the centre level
counseling and home visits are made. Besides, BOCAIP funds outreach
educational programs in the form of emergency material assistance to
needy people infected and affected by HIV and AIDS and is engaged in
orphan care (Maun and Molepolole), support groups for people living with
HIV and AIDS and youth programs (BOCAIP 2008:1). BOCAIP's
activities include, among others, "counseling both pre-test and post-test
and HIV testing; supporting people living with HIV and AIDS; offering
day care facilities for orphaned children; promoting a morally centred
approach to prevention; abstinence and faithfulness; community outreach
to schools and the community at large with a focus on the girl child
education and fight against violence against women and girls; training for
counselors; and referral of clients for further support" (Nkomazana
2007:56). This organization was sub-contracted by Pathfinder International
through PEPFAR and involved peer mothers who are trained to recruit
expecting mothers into the program and provide ongoing psycho-social
support and follow up (NACA 2007:18).

BOCAIP has also been involved in the Youth HIV Prevention and
Blood Safety Project. This project was launched by the Ministry of Health
in November 2003 in order to promote behavior change and HIV
prevention among young people. It was implemented in 2004 by the

Botswana Family Welfare Association (BOFWA), Botswana Christian AIDS Intervention Program (BOCAIP) and the Youth Health Organization (YOHO) with financial support from the African Comprehensive HIV and AIDs Partnerships (ACHAP). The project uses the "Pledge 25 Club" strategy, which involves recruiting young blood donors and encouraging those who are HIV-negative to retain their status. It is estimated that so far a total of 1,432 young people have been reached through this project and that of these 1, 186 (83%) are in –school youth while the remaining 246 comprising (27%) are out-of-school youth. Seventy-six of the out of school youth and 452 in-school youth have pledged to regularly donate blood (NACA 2007:16).

Care of people living with HIV and AIDS through youth initiatives

Another ecumenical effort in the fight against HIV and AIDs in Botswana has been waged by the Youth Psycho-social Initiative. This youth-run psycho-social initiative is a coalition of four churches in Gaborone namely Anglican, Church of the Nazarene, Roman Catholic Church and the Salvation Army. It was formed in April 2002. The Salvation Army Psychological Social Support (SAPSSI) has 800 registered children and a reach of about 3,000 children throughout the country. The centre has both a manual and electronic resource centre which provides children of all school going age with access to the internet and World Wide Web on their door step. The same premise runs a day care/pre-school facility for children in the 2 to 5 year age group. This demonstrates a service that carries children from a very young age to their adolescent years. It has been observed that this service enables care givers at home to become gainfully employed or economically active in some way or another that they may not have if they were providing full time care to infants. The program aims to address the psycho-social issues faced by children who have been left either orphaned or vulnerable as a result of HIV and AIDS. In their dealings with the children the SAPSSI uses the physical, emotional, spiritual and social approach method of education since it sees it as essential to the development of children. This method provides holistic support that is needed by growing children (NACA 2007:27).

The establishment of day care centres in the fight against HIV and AIDS

Apart from the above measures, FBOs have reverted to the method of establishing day care centres in the fight against the HIV and AIDS scourge. Here we shall give some examples from the Roman Catholic Church and the Anglican Church in Botswana. One of the churches in Botswana that has exerted individual efforts in the fight against HIV and AIDS is the Roman Catholic Church. The church began by launching a program called Education for Life. Since the introduction of this program in 2002 more than 1,000 youth have been reached. The objectives of the program are (a) to promote Christian values that enhance peoples' lives and help them live to the fullest; (b) to experience education for life as a process of growth through a journey of conversion and (c) to change behaviour that might put individuals at risk of acquiring HIV and AIDS. The program focuses on behaviour change on the understanding that this would help the individual and the community to reflect on their values, attitudes and life styles. This would, in turn, enable them to make informed responsible choices that can bring positive change. The program is sustained through workshops during which people are encouraged to change their behaviour as the most effective way of combating the epidemic. Participants at such workshops are helped to acquire skills and language that can assist them to break the silence surrounding the epidemic and be able to discuss freely the attitudes, values and behaviour that contribute to the spread of the virus and how to avoid being infected. Education for Life program discourages people from using condoms as the saying goes "Use common sense not condom sense" (Nkomazana 2007:556).

Apart from this program, the Roman Catholic Church also runs a second program called Tirisanyo Catholic Commission. This program addresses, among other things, human rights and social responsibility of both individuals and the voiceless with special focus on the poor, orphans, the disabled and people living with or affected by the HIV and AIDS pandemic. Additionally, the church runs three home-based care programmes in Mogoditshane, Mesimotlhabe and Mompane. Besides, the church runs day care centres for orphans, some of whom are infected, in Tsolamosese, Metsimotlhabe and Thamaga (Nkomazana 2007:56). Services provided in the home based care include (a) daily home visits to patients homes; (b) encouraging clients to go for HIV testing; (c) transporting patients daily for check-ups and visits to VCTs; (d) feeding the infected twice a week; (e) monthly provision of groceries to some patients when funds are available; (f) ensuring supply of food to very weak patients and (g) spiritual counselling every Friday. Apart from the above programs, the Church also runs what is called Games for Life. It targets primary level children. Its objectives are (a) to give children accurate facts on HIV and AIDS and other AIDS related issues in a manner that is culturally applicable and relevant; (b) to give children an opportunity to explore the ways in which they can stay healthy and develop attitudes to cope with outside forces and pressures; (c) to help children develop positive attitudes towards those who are infected and affected by HIV and AIDS and (d) to train leaders and groups of students through the program, who in turn will be able to go out and teach others (Kebakile, Interview).

Another example of day care centres can be drawn from the Anglican Church, which has also been fully involved in the fight against HVI and AIDS for a very long time. Responses from the Anglican Church have been in the form of sermons, seminars and workshops. At the community level the church has established two day care centres and a hospice. One of the centres was established at St. Peters' Church Mogoditshane through the efforts of the resident priest Fr. Andrew Mudereri and his wife Gladys Mudereri. Having seen the plight of children, who had lost their parents and being cared for by their grandmothers, aunts, and some members of the extended family, they were touched by the message of Christ as recorded in Mt.25:31-46, which teaches people to care for those who are in need. They were also moved by the appeal made by the former President Festus Mogae who in 1999 appealed to the nation with the words "Ntwa e boletse! Rise and take your place in the fight against HIV and AIDS." According to Gladys Mudereri, the call of Christ and the President's appeal became a burning fire in their hearts to do what was within their power and capability. Having shared their views with the congregation some people felt drawn to do the work of mercy and compassion. The work needed to be done especially for those children whose caregivers were working and they were left alone at home the whole day. Hence a day care centre and not an orphanage (Mudereri, interview).

St. Peter's Day care Centre was opened on the 1st June 2003 with an initial number of 7 orphans and vulnerable children with the help of five volunteers. By the end of the year they had 11 children two of which were living with HIV and AIDS. By the end of 2004 the number increased to 26. By the end of 2008 the number swelled to 90 children aged between 2.5 and 6 years. The program runs from 7.00 AM until 4.30 PM. The Day Care Centre provides a number of services. It (a) provides psychosocial care (mental, social, physical, emotional and spiritual care) and support to the children and the caregivers; (b) provides quality age appropriate pre-school education to the children; (c) provides nutritional meals throughout the day and (d) monitors the children's weight, height and general health. Children are given breakfast, mid-morning snack, lunch and afternoon snack before they are taken back home. They are given a chance to learn through play and the older ones are prepared for formal school (Mudereri, Interview). A similar Day Care Centre is run by the Anglican Mother's Union in Mahalapye.

The establishment of hospices to alleviate the suffering of the terminally ill

Another way in which the churches have participated in the fight against HIV and AIDS is through the establishment of hospices. A hospice is an organized programme that upon informed choice provides palliative care to terminally ill patients and supportive services to patients, their families and others in both home and facility based services. Physical, social, spiritual and emotional care is provided during the dying process and during bereavement by a medically directed interdisciplinary team consisting of clients, families and volunteers. One such hospice is the Holy Cross Hospice which was founded in 1994. It started as part of the ministry of the Anglican Cathedral in Gaborone and since then it has devoted itself to caring for persons affected by long term and life limiting illnesses such as HIV and AIDS and cancer. In 1995, the Holy Cross began serving patients and their families in Gaborone and Tlokweng by providing home-based physical, emotional and spiritual care services. When it began its services, the hospice focused on home-based care for patients released from Princess Marina Hospital in Gaborone. This was before antiretroviral therapy was introduced and the government initiated community home-based care program. Over the years the hospice has grown from an informal partnership between two nurses and the community into a well trained and highly qualified team of nurses, social workers, community members, as well as local and international volunteers.

It should be noted that palliative care is the core of the hospice's strategic objectives. Located at the Loratong Day Care Centre, the hospice provides HIV and AIDs patients with many forms of medical attention and support. The nurses at the centre provide total nursing care to the patients as well as giving them the necessary medical supplements, monitoring their conditions and offering health education. The nurses also arrange appointments at other health facilities such as the ARV clinics, provide them with transport and escorts for reviews with specialists and conduct follow up visits with patients who are discharged from the centre. A doctor visits the hospice weekly to assess patients and prescribe necessary medications. The doctor also offers medical advice and guidance to the nursing staff. The hospice also provides physical rehabilitation, psychosocial support, and space for a network of staff, volunteers and patients. There is also an effective support group for discharged patients which provides them with a social network and teaches them practical skills to use as a means of generating income if they are unable to find work. Apart from providing services at the Loratong Day care Centre, the hospice also provides Home care to the terminally ill who are too sick to come to the centre. Other patients have caregivers at home who work under the guidance and support of nurses and social work departments. The program focuses on pain and symptom control and management as well as communication with the City Council social workers. In addition to in-home visits, many patients receive meals prepared by the hospice's kitchen staff and are regularly delivered by the hospice drivers. Finally, it should also be noted that the hospice provides care services to orphans and vulnerable children aged 3-18 years through a Pre-School and a Kids Club (Holy Cross Report, no date: 1-3).

Mobilization of the masses through national-wide conferences

As part of the campaign against HIV and AIDS the ecumenical community spearheaded by the Botswana Council of Churches has from time to time hosted activities designed to mobilise public opinion in a grand scale. In this vein, in 2003 a summit was organised jointly by the Botswana Council of Churches, the Evangelical Fellowship of Botswana and the Organisation of African Independent Churches (Southern Region) in which the author served as a resource person. These three national ecumenical organisations in Botswana declared an all out war against HIV and AIDS which has been decimating the population of Botswana and retarding the spiritual, social, economic and political development of the country. The primary purpose of the summit was to enable the churches to reflect theologically and critically on the negative impact that the epidemic was having in the country and to look for ways and means of combating this dreaded epidemic. The theme of the summit was "Come let us rebuild" (Nehemiah 2:17). In itself the theme was an urgent call for Batswana to wake up spiritually and pick up the broken pieces of the Botswana social fabric which has been battered by the HIV and AIDS pandemic in the past twenty four years and once again rebuild the nation and bring it to its former glory. The participants at the summit took cognizance of the fact that the fight against HIV and AIDS needed an ecumenical action if they were to succeed at all. The objectives of the summit were to (a) reflect on the HIV and AIDS situation in Botswana from a faith perspective, (b) to hear what is already happening in the community, (c) to outline the major challenges and problems in the fight against HIV and AIDs, (d) to explore possible areas of cooperation and support and (e) to reflect on a common programme of action and how best to implement such a programme.

At the end of the summit it was strongly recommended that individuals, churches, the community at large, government departments (local and central) as well as the international community should take a daring lead in the fight against the epidemic. At the individual level it was recommended that people should be prepared to go for voluntary testing so that they can know their HIV status and that if they are negative they should strive to remain so and prevent themselves from being infected. An appeal was made to people to abide to biblical ethical principles on matters of sex. Those who are HIV positive were encouraged to live positively and avoid infecting others. The summit advocated behaviour change. People were encouraged to acquire knowledge of HIV and AIDS basic facts, to break communication barriers at all levels, to share knowledge, experiences and government programs available with family, friends and community, acquire knowledge of the psychosexual development of a human being; accept, love, care and support the infected and affected families and create space to share with neighbours and community.

At the ecclesiastical level, the churches were encouraged to work together as a united body of Christ. They were urged to care spiritually, physically, economically, and emotionally those who are affected and infected. It was noted that the churches must take seriously the responsibility to teach the word of God to comfort and encourage members and non-members to embrace biblical ethical principles on matters of human sexuality; be sympathetic with the infected and affected; build trust among the people and provide mental, social and economic care for those in need.

At the community level, the summit called upon Botswana society to critically examine its cultural values with great urgency to avoid the collapse of the entire society. A call was made to uphold monogamous marriage values; encourage abstinence before marriage; impose big penalties for men who impregnate girls before marriage; put an end to the practice of multiple partners; avoid unsafe circumcision methods; discourage co-habitation; condemn incest practices; critically examine cultural cleansing practices; and put an end to men's domineering nature. The Botswana society was also called upon to uphold good aspects of Tswana culture; encouraging partners to go for voluntary testing before marriage; discourage girls from engaging themselves in prostitution and strengthen the values of the extended family in order to be able to care for the sick, the poor, widows and orphans in the community.

At the governmental level, a call was made for the traditional leaders to be empowered with skills that can enable them to mobilize their communities by encouraging traditional leaders to attend seminars, workshops and conferences that deal with HIV and AIDS issues. Traditional leaders were called upon to assess traditional cultural values that promote the spread of HIV and AIDS. A plea was made to the local governments to allocate land for the purpose of building recreation centres such as churches, youth centres, women's empowerment clubs, burial societies and curb activities such as beer feats and others which promote public indecency. The central Government was called upon to consider the issue of couples living apart due to work conditions and outlaw movies that promote promiscuity, passion killings, and that it should make pre-marital counselling compulsory.

Finally the summit looked into the educational system prevalent in the country and recommended that the churches must be involved in the formulation of syllabi for religious and moral education at all levels from primary to university level. It was recommended that HIV and AIDS programs must be injected into the school curricula in order to impart knowledge to students regarding the factors that contribute towards the spread of the epidemic in the country. It was also recommended that all teachers must include in their teaching aspects of the HIV and AIDS pandemic and not only those who teach religious and moral education courses (Amanze and Molefi 2005:4, 91-94).

Ethical considerations lead to strong opposition against the use of condoms

It has been noted above that the link between the HIV and AIDS pandemic with sexual activity led to the moralisation of the epidemic. This was evident especially when the government advocated that one way of fighting against the pandemic was the use of condoms. This message did not augur well among the FBOs. They accused the government and medical practitioners of encouraging and promoting immorality among the Botswana population. The use of condoms escalated in the mid 1990s. Since 1993, the Population Services International (PSI) has helped to promote the 'Lovers Plus' condoms and since 2002 the 'care' female condom. One of PSI's key strategies for marketing condoms has been peer education, which has been conducted in a variety of settings such as fairs and festivals, shopping malls, workplaces and bars. In 2003 the government of Botswana, with funding and technical support from ACHAP, launched an extensive condom distribution and marketing campaign, providing for the installation of 10,500 dispensers in traditional and non-traditional outlets throughout the country. Millions of condoms have been procured for free distribution (http://www.avert.org/aids botswana.htm). This is an area that FBOs have opposed very strongly. The majority of FBOs in Botswana reject the idea of condomising by Christians, especially those who are not married, on the understanding that condoms will only promote promiscuity. It is strongly believed that Christians must believe in the saving power of God and that if they abstain and stick to one partner they will be delivered from the present scourge. Christians, it is argued, should never give up their role of being "The Light of the World" and the "Salt of the World" in an era of moral degradation. Therefore, it is maintained, it is morally wrong for the churches to support and encourage people to use condoms in all circumstances. It is argued in certain quarters that it is better for a Christian to have unprotected sex and face the consequences rather than using condoms and pretend before God and the Church that one is holy. The use of condoms, it is argued, is sinful hence equally punishable by God who detests sin and any form of immorality.

Full circle? Churches come to terms with reality: Ban on condom use lifted

It has been noted above that while other means of preventing the HIV and AIDS scourge are acceptable by all member churches of the BCC, there has been a growing concern regarding the use of condoms by Christians as advised by health service providers. For a long time, therefore, the BCC has discouraged people from using condoms on the understanding that the use of condoms promotes immorality and that condoms do not provide 100% protection to those who use them. There has also been great opposition towards the idea of promoting and distributing condoms to the under-aged youth through the school system. However, because of the severity of the scourge, the BCC decided to take a U-turn and accept the idea that, though condoms are not an ideal form of combating HIV and AIDS, they can, nonetheless, serve as preventative mechanisms. With this in mind, at the 34th Annual Assembly, it was resolved that the fight against the HIV and AIDS pandemic should include the following: the teaching of Religious and Moral Education in schools, empowerment and holding of community education on HIV and AIDS through workshops, seminars and other effective channels. Furthermore the use of condoms should be encouraged only as an alternative where people cannot abstain (Amanze 2006:221).

Concluding Remarks

This chapter has discussed the role played by the FBOs in the fight against the HIV and AIDS pandemic in Botswana. The chapter began by examining the theology of the Christian churches on human sexuality and has concluded that their understanding is that human sexuality is a gift from God and that it must be used responsibly. It has been noted that the fact that the spread of the HIV and AIDS pandemic is linked with human sexuality in many aspects of its manifestation led to stigma and discrimination of people living with HIV and AIDS. This led to the slow pace at which Faith Based Organisations reacted to the situation in order to reduce the suffering of PLWHA and bring normality to the situation. Different strategies adopted by the FBOs in the struggle against HIV and AIDS have been discussed. All in all, it can be concluded that FBOs have contributed tremendously in the fight against the epidemic and that they have been a true partner in the struggle to emancipate the Botswana nation from the throes of death and annihilation.

Bibliography

Amanze, J. N. "Covenant with death: The attitude of the churches in Botswana towards the use of condoms by Christians and its social implications", *Botswana Notes and Records,* Vol.32, 2000, .201-208.
—. *Botswana handbook of Churches,* Gaborone: Pula Press, 1994.
—. "Stigma: The greatest obstacle in the fight against HIV/AIDS in Africa" in J. N. Amanze et al (eds.), *Christian Ethics and HIV/AIDS in Africa,* Gaborone: Bay Publishing, 2007, 28-47.
Amanze, J. N. & Molefi, K, (eds.), *Church and HIV/AIDS,* Gaborone: Botswana Council of Churches, 2005.
Amanze, J. N. *Ecumenism in Botswana: The Story of the Botswana Christian Council,* Gaborone: Pula Press, 2006.
ASRH-Adolescents Sexual Reproductive Health, a pamphlet of the Botswana Council of Churches (no date)
BCC, Minutes of the Executive Committee of the BCC, May 1993.

—. *Mokaedi:,* monthly newsletter of the Botswana Christian Council, Gaborone, 5ᵗʰ March 2003.

BOCAIP, http://bocaip.org/activities.htm.

Flannery, A. (ed.), *Vatican Council* II, New York: Liturgical Press, 1982.

HIV and AIDS in Botswana, http://www.avert.org/aidsbotswana.htm, accessed on 11/12/2008

Holy Cross Hospice Report to 2008 Vision 2016 Awards (no date). http://www.globalhealthreporting.org/countries/Botswanana.asp.

Mogomotsi, B. W. "Efforts towards HIV/AIDS prevention-the case of Botswana" paper presented at the workshop on Learning and empowerment: Key issues in strategies for HIV/AIDS prevention held in Chiangmai, Thailand, March 2004.

National AIDS Coordinating Agency, *Progress Report of the national Response to the UNGASS Declaration of Commitment on HIV/AIDS,* Ministry of State President, December 2007.

Nkomazana, F. "Christian Ethics and HIV/AIDS in Botswana", in J. N. Amanze Et al (eds.), *Christian Ethics and HIV/AIDS in Africa,* Gaborone: Bay Publishing, 2007, 48-69.

Parry, S. *Responses of the Faith Based Organisations to HIV/AIDS in Sub-Saharan Africa,* World Council of Churches, Geneva: 2003.

The New Penguin English Dictionary, London: Penguin Books, 2000.

"Tirisanyo Catholic Commission, Progress Report on HIV/AIDS from January to August 2004, pp.1-5.

World Council of Churches Statement on churches compassionate response to HIV and AIDS, September 2006.

Interviews

Bothongo, Bishop Peterson, Interview, Gaborone, 22/10/1999.

Cloete, Rev. Arthur. Interview, Gaborone, 22/9/199.

Corrigan, Fr. John, Interview, Gaborone, 23/10/1999.

Habibo, Rev. Raphael. Interview, Gaborone, 10/10/1999.

Hambira, Rev. Rupert, Interview, Gaborone, 11/10/1999.

Kebakile, Sister Angela (Coordinator of HIV and AIDS in the Diocese of Gaborone), Interview, Gaborone, 6/1/2009.

Kwarapi, Rev. Johannes, Interview, Gaborone, 11/10/1999.

Makhulu Archbishop A. K. (former Bishop of the Diocese of Botswana), Interview, Gaborone, 12/10/99.Mere, Rev. O. E. Interview, Gaborone, 26/9/1999.

Modiega, David (General Secretary of the Botswana Council of Churches), Interview, Gaborone, 24/10/2004.

Mpofu, Pastor A. Interview, Mogoditshane, 2/10/1999.
Mudereri, Gladys (Centre Manager), Interview, Mogoditshane, 6/1/2009.
Ntuping, Bishop M. Interview, Gaborone, 16/91999.
Robinson, Bishop J. Interview, Gaborone, 18/9/1999.

PART IV:

RELIGION AND CULTURE

CHAPTER ELEVEN

NTWA E BOLOTSE:
BOTSWANA WOMEN, MEN AND HIV/AIDS[1]

MUSA W. DUBE

Ntwa e Bolotse (The War Has Started):
Can We Fight Back?

In the war against HIV and AIDS, the African continent is in the midst of the storm, since we host 67% of the 36 million people living with HIV and AIDS in Sub-Saharan Africa (UNAIDS, 2008:7). Many of us have lived long enough to remember the African struggle for political liberation. Some of you might thus agree that it was only yesterday, when we were fighting for our liberation from colonial oppression. The songs of the struggle for liberation are still ringing in our ears. Indeed it was only yesterday that the beautiful feet of lady liberation touched the mountains of the African continent, announcing the good news of peace and salvation. And just as a smile was on our faces, as we heard the sweet sound of lady liberation coming down to dwell with us, there was another big bang. Africa was struck by another oppressor: HIV and AIDS. We are back to the battlefield, fighting for our liberation, again. Thus we have to take our place in the battle against HIV and AIDS and become effective foot soldiers.

As soldiers in the war against HIV and AIDS, we cannot afford to be ignorant about how our enemy creeps on us and the ladders it uses to climb in. Extensive information and educational campaigns and research have been carried out worldwide. One of the major drivers of the epidemic

---

[1] An earlier version of this paper was published as "Culture, Gender and HIV/AIDS: Understanding and Acting on the Issues," in   Musa W. Dube, eds. *HIV/AIDS and the Curriculum: Methods of Integrating HIV/AIDS in Theological Programs.* Geneva: WCC. The second version is produced here with permission from the publisher.

that we cannot afford to ignore in the fight against HIV and AIDS is gender inequality. Research indicates that "gender inequalities are a major driving force behind the AIDS epidemic" (UNAIDS, 2000:21). If we are going to be part of the solution in seeking to reduce and finally eradicate the spread and impact of HIV and AIDS in the African continent and our particular countries, we must fully understand gender inequalities. The *Botswana Human Development Report* (2000), consequently emphasized that "the starting point for an adequate response is the understanding that any bid to halt the AIDS epidemic has to include determined efforts to eradicate poverty and to drastically reduce inequalities" (2000:56). The link between gender inequalities and vulnerability is consistently attested. For example, *The Botswana AIDS Impact Survey II (BAIS II)* of 2004 found that "in terms of gender the sharpest differences were recorded among those between 15 and 29, with 10% of the females and only 3% of the males aged between 15-19 being HIV positive" (quoted in NACA 2004:5). The recently released *BAIS III*, also shows vulnerability to HIV infection along gender lines. "The 2008 *Botswana AIDS Impact Survey III (BAIS III)* data yielded a national prevalence rate of 17.6 percent... by gender the prevalence among females was 20.4 percent while males had 14.2 percent. The rate of new infections was higher among females than males at an estimated 3.5 and 2.3 percent respectively (*The Midweek Sun, Ghetto Metro*, Wednesday June 3, 2009: ii). "Worldwide HIV and AIDS research indicates that "gender-based inequalities overlap with other social, cultural, economic and political inequalities—and affect women and men of all ages" (UNAIDS 2000: 21). Clearly, "literature indicates that the spread of the epidemic affects the health of men and women differently, depending on their age, class, sexual orientation" (Shaibu and Dube 2002:5).

When the then president of Botswana, Mr Festus Mogae, launched the national struggle against HIV and AIDS; when he officially declared HIV and AIDS as a national emergency that should be tackled by government, private and civil society sectors; by individuals and families; by communities and nations, he declared, *"Ntwa e bolotse,"* that is, we are in a warfare (BNSF 2003:15). The question for all of us then is, can we pick our guns, position ourselves and get ready to do battle with HIV and AIDS? It is a different warfare. The enemy today is hardly outside our continents; it is hardly outside our countries; it is hardly outside our families; it is hardly outside our bodies. One sometimes wishes the enemy was over there, so we could identify it, take cover or shoot it down and be done with it. But, lo and behold, our worst enemy is amongst us and in us. It is everywhere. It is between men and women; it is between boys and girls; it is between husbands and wives; it is between lovers of all sexual orientations; it is in the beds of our intimacy—in the best moments of our lives--when we kiss and make love. Lo and behold, the enemy is there. The enemy is now in our veins: in our blood, in our cells, in our fluids, in our minds. HIV makes love with us; drags and drugs us to death. The quest is thus quite poignant: Can we pick our guns, position ourselves and get ready to do battle with HIV and AIDS? The battle call has long been sounded when the former President of Botswana, Mr F. Mogae, declared that, *"Ntwa e bolotse."*

We are, therefore, back to the battlefield, fighting for our liberation again. The big question, I repeat, is: are we ready to do battle against HIV and AIDS? Are we ready to take our guns and shoot? This warfare requires different rules from us. It requires all of us as women and men to interrogate ourselves; to admit that we are part of the problem and to change some of the dearest aspects of our lives. It requires us to interrogate the very things that we have always taken for granted. It requires us to interrogate our frames of reference, our values, our ways of life. It requires us to admit that these need to change and that no one will change them for us, but rather we must change them ourselves!!!! I can by no means glamorize the task at hand—it is a complicated struggle. It is therefore a sobering moment, a critical moment, for we have to shoot at a very close enemy that lives among us and in us. We have to look much closely, close, at home, at ourselves and interrogate our relationships and all those things that we do that promote the spread of HIV and AIDS.

There are many HIV and AIDS drivers such as poverty, risky behavior, alcohol abuse, violence and stigma and discrimination. In this chapter, I seek to focus on one of the major drivers of HIV and AIDS; namely, gender inequalities. As said, in the battle against the HIV epidemic we cannot afford to be ignorant about how our enemy moves and creeps in and among us as individuals, families, communities and our nations. One of the factors that we need to understand in this struggle for liberation is gender: What is gender? What sustains gender? How does religion and culture construct and maintain gender? Why is gender a major factor in the spread of HIV and AIDS and how can we shoot down the gender inequalities? This chapter seeks to address these questions in their given order.

What is Gender?

Gender is a social construction of men and women. Geeta Rao Gupta describes gender as "a culture –specific construct" (2000:1). S/he goes on to break this down by saying, "there are significant differences in what women and men can do or cannot do in one culture as compared to one another. But it is fairly consistent across cultures" (2000:1). Before we proceed to look at the details of what these differences entail, let me pause here to underline a few things. First, the fact that gender is culturally constructed needs to be underlined. This means that gender:

- is not natural
- is not divine
- has to do with social relationships of women and men
- can be reconstructed and transformed by the society for it is culturally constructed, hence it can be socially deconstructed.

I must also return to an earlier quote; namely that gender overlaps with "other social, cultural, economic and political" factors. In short, gender is a complex issue that works with and through all social departments. The fact that gender overlaps with the social, cultural, economical, and political departments of our lives underlines that—gender pervades all aspects of our lives. Gender, if I may make a literal translation, is everything and it is everywhere. We are, in other words, always socially constructed as men and women in our various cultures, in our politics, in our governments, in our schools, in our villages, in our cities, in our workplaces, in our homes, in our conversations, in our beds—making love!! We are always socially constructed.

The way we relate in all these relationships, at all the times, and at all places is "always gendered," that is, it is always socially constructed. It is always according to the dictates or within the frameworks of what is socially expected from us as women and men. Think of the way you eat, the way you dress; think of the perfume you wear, the sock, the shoe, your hair style. Are they the same for women and men? Well those are the obvious ones. I can very well say, "think of the way you think, the way you feel, the way you taste, the way you see, the way you hear... all that if you think it is as natural as water, it is not. Even the way you feel, see, hear, taste, and smell is gendered—it is a product of social construction. Take, for example, how we may feel pain or not feel it. Men have been constructed to take it like a man—that is, 'don't ever cry unless your heart is going to break.' So men are socially constructed not to express their feelings of fear and pain. They are to be fearless and brave. They are not to show emotions. Women, on the other hand, are socially constructed to cry, to express their feelings, to be timid and fearful, and many times—they are not supposed to think. Even when they think, what they think is

supposed to be interpreted as senseless. So what is so natural about crying
when you feel pain or not crying? I am touching on these to highlight that
gender is a complex and deeply embedded socialization and that none of
us have escaped its construction. We are gendered human beings, all the
time, everywhere. The best we can do is to be critically aware of our
gendered perspectives and identities.

Gender construction is hegemonic in the sense that it pervades all
aspects of our lives and all aspects of our human senses so much so that
many of us are likely to think that it is natural and many times we think it
is divine—hence unchangeable. This is the strength and difficulty of
dealing with gender issues; namely, that many people think that gender is
natural or biological. It is not. Gender is a social product; hence we the
members of the society can reconstruct it, if and when we find it wanting.
For example, for the people of our era, we have been brought to realize
that gender is "a major driving force behind the AIDS epidemic"
(UNAIDS 2000: 21). This, I insist, is more than enough reason for us to
seek to change our current gender construction.

The Problem with Gender Construction

Let us pause and ask one question: That is, if both women and men are
gendered, why does this bother us? Why should we be looking at the
issues of gender and culture?   Perhaps our question should be: why has
gender become "a major driving force" behind the spread of HIV and
AIDS? Gupta's explication of gender is useful here. Gupta says, in gender

> there is always a distinct difference between women's and men's roles,
> access to productive resources outside the home and decision-making
> authority. Typically, men are seen as being responsible for the productive
> activities outside the home while women are expected to be responsible for
> reproductive and productive activities within the home...women have less
> access over control of productive resources than men—resources such as
> income, land, credit, and education, (2000:2).

In short, gender construction does not distribute power equally between
men and women.   Men are constructed as public leaders, thinkers,
decision-makers and property owners. Women are constructed primarily
as domestic beings, those who belong to the home or the kitchen, the
mothers, wives. They are constructed to be dependent on the property of
their husbands, brothers or fathers. Women are constructed to be silent,
non-intelligent, emotional, well behaved, non-questioning, obedient,
faithful to one partner—be they fathers, husbands, boyfriends or live-in

partners. And so we think of a good woman as one who takes a very good care of her home, children, husband, one who hardly questions or speaks back to her partner and one who remains faithful to their partner. A good man is one who is fearless, brave, property owner, public leader, and in some cultures, he is one who may have more than one sexual partner.

At the center of gender relations is the concept of power and powerlessness. The problem is that gender construction dis-empowers half of humanity—the women folk. It is on these grounds that Ally Purvis says "women are not subjects in the same way that men are. A woman is a derivative concept that exists only as an object of a man's attention," (1995:125). This dire discrepancy in the distribution of power is becoming our unmaking in the HIV and AIDS era. It is the fertile ground upon which the virus thrives—women who are constructed as powerless cannot insist on safer sex, for the decision lies with a man. They can hardly abstain for sexual violence is another instrument that men use to forcefully take women's bodies (Botswana Police Report 1999). Similarly, faithfulness does not guarantee partners from HIV infection, especially the married women. Men who have been constructed to be fearless, brave, and sometimes reckless, think it is a manly thing to do when they refuse to heed the warning that unprotected sex can lead them to HIV infection. Working within the cultural allowance of extra-marital affairs, Batswana men continue to have extra-marital relations—at the end no one wins. We all die: those with power and those without power. I am sure you will agree that there is no point in keeping such gender constructions. In the HIV and AIDS context, no one is served, save for the virus that finds easy inroads within the fault lines of gender constructions. It's unfair distribution of power is a poison in our plate—the wicked and deadly witch. I am sure you will want us to exorcise the wicked power of gender inequalities within our families and communities.

It is important to remember that gender construction takes on many other social factors. It works together with economy, politics, and culture. Gender works with other social factors such as class, ethnicity, race, age, physical challenge and sexual orientation. It varies from one group to another. The way a particular race and ethnic group constructs gender will be different from how others do it—but one constant thing has been found—access to resources, decision making and public leadership are not equally distributed amongst men and women. For example, the English say, "ladies first," meaning men have to come behind so the men can protect the supposedly weak women. Other cultures do not say ladies first, in fact, the man walks in front and the woman comes from behind. For example, the Batswana say *"Ga dinke dietelelwa ke tse di namagadi,"* meaning women, must follow men. In both thinking, of ladies first and ladies behind, the man is constructed as the brave one and the leader while the woman is constructed as the weak one, the one to be protected and the one to follow the leader. Similarly, some cultures speak of polyandry and others speak of polygamy, yet a close study has shown that matriarchal cultures are by no means woman centered than patriarchal ones (Oduyoye 1986:122). In short, gender research reflects that in most cultures the balance of power bends towards the male folk than women folk.

Gender Construction and Maintenance: The Case of Botswana Cultures

Culture becomes central to gender when we ask the question: "how is gender constructed and maintained?" Something as deep and as pervasive as gender needs a host of social support systems that convert the mind and the heart, for its own maintenance and reduplication through ages. Gender can only thrive through myth, cultural and religious beliefs that seemingly naturalize and sanctify what is certainly a social construct. I would like us to plot the construction of gender from birth to death by showing how this gender is maintained and reproduced in culture using the case of some African cultures, particularly Setswana cultures. We shall begin by briefly defining culture and then move to plot gender construction from birth to death.

Culture and Gender

What is culture? This is a very complex word. We cannot deal with all its aspects here. I only wish to give a number of definitions, which shall be central to our analysis. According to Musimbi Kanyoro,

> a particular people (nation, tribe, ethnic group) has its own culture, its distinct way of living, loving, eating, playing and worshiping. Culture may refer to the musical and visual arts, modern influences on life, an acquired tradition, or to regulations that bind the life of a community... Culture can be a double-edged sword: it can form community identity and it can also be used to set apart or oppress those whom culture defines as other. Participation in culture is so natural and ubiquitous that most people take culture for granted (2000:62).

According to Kenneth Surin, culture is "a particular way of life, whether of a people, a period, a group or humanity in general," (2000:49). Culture "refers to the material production of a society," (Colombia Dictionary

1995:66), which becomes a "central system of practices, meanings and values and which we can properly call dominant and effective" (Surin, 2000:51).

One of the most well known definitions of culture is the Marxist one. It holds that culture is a product of the ruling class which serves to keep the powerless dominated. The latter is best exemplified by cultural gender constructions—it is from the male perspective, which is the perspective of those empowered, which hardly benefits the subjugated, the females. The Marxist perspective regards culture, therefore, as an ideology that is formulated by those in power for their own ends. Culture does not serve all members of the society, although it is applied to all. In the Marxist perspective culture therefore is "both materially informed and informing" (Columbia Dictionary, 1995:66). Expounding on this perspective, R. Boer holds that in a Marxist frame, "culture shares space with religion, the state, intellectual endeavor and so on, which are then set over against economics, the relationship being mediated by social class" (1999:169). In the light of contemporary forms of communications "culture has undergone yet another transformation in its usage. We now have a seemingly limitless access to activities, attitudes, and aesthetic ideals that do not necessarily jibe with the assumptions about taste and sensibilities that are promulgates by the standards of a dominant culture" (Columbia Dictionary, 1995: 67). Let us now try to draw some main points from these definitions. We can say that culture:

- Engulfs us all--no one exists outside one or another culture.
- Is a major framework of meaning, which guides how our relationships are formulated and lived out.
- Is different for different people, groups and times, etc.
- Does not always serve the needs and interest of all its members of the society.
- Sanctions the suppression of certain members of the society in the interest of those in power.
- Is not natural, it is a social product.
- Is not static, it is dynamic. It changes.

Inculturation of Gender: From Birth to Death

With this background on culture, let us now turn to the question of how does gender intersect with culture? Is gender the sub-sect of culture or the other way round? I think we can safely say that gender is a cultural product. I will illustrate this point by plotting how gender is socially formulated within a culture from birth to death. I shall draw most of my examples from Setswana cultures, although I will also refer to others.

Birth

We are all born into a society and a culture. What happens when a boy or girl is born? How is gender marked? In most cultures the child is named. The naming can be neutral or gender specific, or both. Naming thus becomes the first social construction. In the Setswana cultures, for example names can be gender-neutral or gender-specific. Gender neutral names are those that are given to both genders such as Tshepo (the trusted one); Thato (God's will), Kelebogile (I am grateful, Mpho (gift). Setswana naming can also be gender-specific. Thus a girl-child might be named as Segametsi (one who draws water); Mosidi (one who grinds flour) Bontle (beauty), Khumo (one who brings bride wealth) Boingotlo (the humble one), Dikeledi (tears, one who cries); Maitseo (the one who behaves well), Lorato (love). Boy children may be given the following names Modisaotsile (the shepherd); Mojaboswa (the inheritor) Kgosi (the leader) Seganka (the brave one). Each one of us can think of their own naming system and scrutinize if it distributes power of leadership, property ownership and public leadership equally amongst boys and girls. In the Setswana naming system, the gender-specific names spell out the gender roles. Gender-specific names do not distribute power equally amongst boys and girls. The boy child is marked as leader, property owner, and public leader. The girl child is a domestic player, a humble one, a lover and one who must be beautiful.

Clothing

A recently acquired culture among Batswana is that a baby boy child is dressed in blue colors. I do not know what blue stands for, but one may well say, blue represents that they must be out of the house in the blue skies. A baby girl, on the other hand, is wrapped in pink colors, perhaps representing a flower, something that must be beautiful and attractive. While I am not sure about the meaning of these colors, the point here is that both the girl and boy child are marked and socially constructed differently at birth even through the colors they wear.

Toys

On top of names and clothes, we construct gender through the toys that we buy our kids or the games that we teach our children. In Setswana cultures, the boys made cows while girls made pots and dolls. We buy cars, airplanes and guns for boys, while for girls we buy coffee sets, beauty sets or baby dolls. These toys are quite consistent with the names that associate boys with property/cattle (Modisaotsile) and girl with domestic roles (Segametsi).

Role Modeling

Children learn their gender roles most powerfully from their parents. They are watching what the Father is doing and what the Mother is doing. Soon you will find them playing the home (*mmantlwane*) on their own and you will be surprised at how precise they have learnt gender roles. Here children absorb culture and gender roles through informal education of observing their parents and neighbors. One time, when I was moving house, I heard my young sister's five year old son saying, "Me and my Father can lift everything here." Despite that he was five years old, he already believed that whatever his father can lift he can also lift. The boy had already understood that society expects him to be strong by observing what his father does.

Childhood Stage

The childhood stage is characterized by culturally educating what the society expects from them through storytelling, language, proverbs, and school. In Setswana cultures children learnt proverbs and storytelling around the fireplace. If one analyses the sayings, stories and proverbs for what they say about women and men, one finds that it is a cultural bank; a bank that does not distribute power equally amongst different genders. There are such proverbs as "*gandinke di etelelwa ke tse di namagadi* (a woman never leads*) Monna o wa kgomothwa* (a man need not be handsome—just pick any*). Mosadi tshwene o jewa maboga* (a woman's labor is harvested by someone else). In storytelling, children learnt many stories that taught that a good girl is one who is obedient and cooks a good meal for her husband (the two daughters); a girl must care about beauty (Tsananapo); a boy must care about cows/property (Masilo) and a boy must be a brave protector of women (delele). While indigenous ways of socializing children into accepted roles has been overtaken by urbanization and western media, the gendering is still quite prevalent in TV programs—the video games, the movies and soap operas that our children watch and the magazines that they read. Brian Wren points out that,

Many films center on male characters, with whom the viewer is invited to identify, and on sexuality as pursuit. Men pursue women, whether in love or lust, crude dominance or tender possession.... We who are watching (tacitly assumed to be "we men") are meant to find pleasure in seeing a woman in peril, and the excitement at her vulnerability and terror... We are encouraged to take the male role of superiority ("we'd do better than that") and indulge our desire to rape and conquer, or protect and rescue... Sometimes the male viewer is encouraged into the position of a rapist in relation to the woman. We can see her, but she can't see us. Though that is true of film and TV as a medium, it is often played on sexually (1989: 18).

Formal School

The school plays a similar role in the gender construction of children. The contents of school textbooks reproduce the same cultural gender roles. Pictures will feature the Mother going to the market to buy vegetables, while the Father goes to take care of cattle. Textbooks consistently feature men sitting at the Kgotla (village court), hence underlining that leadership is a man's role. Pictures and contents of the books that school-going children read thus endorse gender roles that are propounded in the general culture. Although these days it is a subject of much scrutiny, a lot still needs to be done.

Teenage and Adulthood

In Setswana traditional cultures, boys and girls were taken to circumcision schools that marked their growth from children to adulthood. In these schools, gender roles were culturally taught. Boys were taught what it means to be a man and girls were equably instructed on what the culture expects from them as women (Schapera 1938: 104-118). Boys' initiation school was called *Bogwera*, while *Bojale* was for the girls. Boys were instructed that manhood involved frequent attendance of the *kgotla* (court), readiness to fight and protect the society, rearing and loving cattle, responsible sexuality, the duty to marry and maintain a family. The teenage girls were taught that responsible womanhood included taking care of agricultural production, building houses/home, maintaining the Kgosi (community leader) home, maintenance of one's marriage and raising children. Professionally, both boys/men and girls/women were allocated career roles (cattle-rearing for men and agriculture for women), public leadership and law-making leaned towards men.

Marriage

This stage is one of those rites of passage where gender roles are underlined and reinforced. In Setswana cultures, the old women take the new bride and counsel her quite painfully until she cries. Some of the things they say include: *tlogela ditsala* (you must give up your friends and focus on your marriage); *"nyalo e a itshokelwa"* (you must endure marriage, it will be difficult). *Ngwanaka, monna ga a botswe kwa a tswang* (my child, a man is never asked where he went or slept). *Monna phafana oa fapanelwa* (a man is a calabash of beer that is passed around); *Monna poo ga agelwe lesaka* (a man is a bull who must not be confined to one kraal, or should be free to move around and see other women outside his marriage kraal). Some of the sayings indicate that Setswana culture expects and tolerates a married man's unfaithfulness and does not see it as a good reason for divorce. Some of the advices include, "You must remember that the path to a man's heart is food," that is, cook for him. "If your husband hits you, and you get a blue eye, never reveal it—rather, say you bumped on the wall on your way to the toilet in the dark." Here violence in institutionally tolerated! The bridegroom, on the other hand, hardly gets any intensified counseling about his role as a husband, partly because married men are married-bachelors. Their canceling is usually brief and outside, where they are told, 'today you are a man. See to it that your wife and children have food and shelter. They should never sleep hungry. Make sure they are protected." In most cases, the new husband is not counseled. It is just assumed he knows what it means to be a husband.

The adumbration of gender roles during marriage and the wedding celebration is also evident in the songs that are sung and the acts that are carried out. One of the most dramatic demonstrations of gender roles in a wedding of the northern Botswana is when the bride enters the home from the church. Guests will stand in two rows holding all the domestic items and acting out what a wife is expected to do. As she walks in, holding the hand of her husband, some will be pounding, some will be weeding, others will be nursing a baby, some will be sweeping, some will be cooking, some will be carrying a bundle of firewood—everything will be demonstrated and all this happens in the middle of great singing, dancing and ululation. Again, in this demonstration of gender roles, very little is said about the role of a husband—except that the husband is to expect all these numerous activities from his wife. Some of the latest gendered traditions surrounding marriage are what they call kitchen parties or bridal showers. The fact that it is called kitchen party, speaks volumes on what is expected from the wife. Yes, there is a bachelor's party and I am sure we have seen on TVs and movies what happens there!

Old Age

In old age women and men are still culturally constructed along gender roles. A man is held to remain a man (you remember Wole Soyinka's story of The Lion and the Jewel?) In fact, a man is fully entitled, in some Setswana cultures, to find a young woman to make his blood to move again (Shaibu & Dube 2002:6). In some of the Botswana cultures the aging wife was responsible for seeking a younger woman for her husband to marry. This gave the first wife some power by bringing a younger woman, who would be loyal to her, often by seeking a relative of hers. The latter cultural belief has translated itself as a deadly practice in the HIV and AIDS era. Elderly men seek young girls/virgins in the hope that they can cleanse themselves of HIV and AIDS. Because they have money, they lure the poor young girls, infect them and move on. Meanwhile young boys seek these young girls and get them infected. This is the so called trans-generational sex. The latter makes the dream of raising an HIV and AIDS free generation difficult. The absolute desperation created by HIV and AIDS, coupled by this belief of rejuvenation means that even girl infants are sometimes subjected to rape by relatives, strangers, neighbors and by their own fathers. Since children are supposedly the "window of hope" in the fight against HIV, these sexual gendered cultural beliefs and practices must be confronted, for they serve as pathways for HIV.

How are elderly and old women constructed? Menopausal women, who may be less interested in sex, are held to be unclean to their husbands. They supposedly do not cleanse the blood of their husband. Consequently, at menopausal stage Setswana indigenous cultures entertained the departure of a husband to find another woman, or authorized the legal wife to find a younger wife. What about the very old women, especially widows and grandmothers? These often get stereotyped as witches. Think of your village, and remember all the women who were rumored to be dangerous witches. They were mostly women, especially very old women. This association of old women with evil has been quite deadly in some of African cultures, especially east Africa, where old women are sought out during the night and hacked to death.

Death

Death does not escape from gender constructions. Many cultures have put in place rituals, which reinforce and maintain gender roles surrounding death. In the event of death of a spouse, in some Botswana and Southern

African cultures, an elder/younger brother was expected to inherit the widow. This cultural practice, which has become less prevalent, is known as *seantlo*. This practice ensured that property is kept with the family of the husband. What does a young man who is supposed to inherit his brother's wife do, if the elder brother died of AIDS and has left behind an infected widow? What about a widow who may not be infected, but has to be inherited by an infected member of the family? It goes without saying that such cultural practices were indeed informed by gender construction that placed property ownership in the hands of men. A widow was thus better inherited for her to retain her social security.

Of late, a widow may be dispossessed by the family of her husband, who are not willing to inherit her and unwilling to allow her to inherit the property of her husband. Dispossession leads some widows to desperation and to engage in survival sex, which does not help in the HIV prevention. In other cultures, such as Botswana ones, widows undergo quite painful rituals to cleanse them of the blood of their dead man. In Botswana a widow must wear a black or blue dress for the whole year to mark her status and warn other men to stay away, for any man who has sexual intercourse with a widow before the cleansing ceremony will supposedly fall ill. During this period, therefore, she must not see another man. The widower, however, does not have to wear black mourning clothes, for the society to know him, although he is expected to undergo ritual cleansing. It follows that a widower does not have to abstain, except out of his own good will towards his late wife.

In Setswana indigenous cultures, burials of women and men were and still are gender marked. A man was buried in a kraal, wrapped in a fresh skin of a cow, and well equipped with weapons of war--his spears and rods. A woman could be buried in the home, with pots and other cooking utensils. The cultural thinking is that even in other life/heaven women and men would still be pursuing their socially ascribed roles. God forbid! In some Batswana cultures once married away from one's ethnic group, a woman cannot return to be buried in her home town/village. That is, a married woman is married—dead or alive.

Maintenance of Gender Roles in Culture

The above plot of cultural construction of gender roles from birth to death underlines the depth of gender constructions in our socialization. Yet it is only a tip of the iceberg. It does not, for example, highlight that gender roles are daily underlined in the languages that we speak, in our laws, jokes and religion. In English language, for example, we find major gender constructions. A young woman who is not married is called a "miss"—one who is missing something. When she marries she then becomes whole, by taking the title of Mrs. If she gets divorced she will become a "miss" again. A man, on the other hand, is a Mr before and after marriage, in divorce and widowhood—he never changes. The words "he" "son" "man" are the root forms of such words like "wo/man" "per/son" "man/kind," "s/he" thus underlining that English culture views the relationships from a male perspective. The male is the subject while the woman is his derivative. To counteract this overt male-oriented language, gender inclusive English language have been coined, such as "Ms instead of Miss"; humankind instead of mankind, chairperson instead of chairman; director of ceremonies instead of master of ceremonies.

Gender roles are also underlined through national laws that do not give equal power to women and men. In Botswana, the in-community of property marriage, for example, reduced the status of a woman to "a minor." This meant that upon marriage, the husband became the property owner and manager of whatever they own and whatever the woman owns or makes. Husbands planning to get a divorce commonly sold all property before filing for divorce, given that their wives' status was that of minors. A married woman could not even get a loan from the bank without her husband's consent, given her status as a minor. In this way, the dependency and desperation of a woman is lawfully maintained. Batswana women's movement fought to get the in-community marriage laws reviewed to include power of attorney to both partners, a stance that restored women's adulthood and debarred husbands from selling property without the consent of their husbands, when they wished to divorce.

Further, the social institutions of the family, the school, the church, village and the parliament and the cabinet, more often than not, underline the cultural gender roles by keeping men as leaders and women as sub-ordinates. How then do we expect girls who grew up under the leadership of a father, a male principal, a male village leader, a male pastor, a male Member of Parliament and male president to suddenly believe in their own capacity to lead or believe in the leadership of other women? And so we have heard and seen it happen in many cases—whenever you give women a chance to choose a leader, they prefer to choose a man than another woman. We see it all the time in public politics, that women are the majority of voters, but they will not use their votes to vote other women into power, instead they vote men into power. Similarly, how do we expect a boy who has grown up in all-male social leadership to accept women leadership? And so many of us can recall how those women who rise in their own institutions to leadership are often stereotyped, rejected and named as cruel iron ladies or queen bees.

Jokes and labels are another cultural instrument used by society to maintain ascribed gender roles. Boys who do not play the hard macho ball; those who demonstrate emotions and emotional feelings are castigated and labeled sissies or dabbed chicken soup. In Setswana, this kind of boy is labeled *pharamesising* (one who sits around dresses). Similarly, a husband who is found cleaning the house, cooking, changing nappies, is most likely to be dismissed as a man who has been duped with love portions, bewitched by his wife and one who badly needs to be helped to vomit the love portions to redeem his masculinity. Girls who do not invest much time on beauty and who show a degree of independence and physical strength are similarly labeled "tom boys.' Women who speak up and express interest in a man of their choice will get labeled as cheap women. Friends, relatives and neighbors throw these jokes and labels, which are actually social instruments that serve to pressurize the deviating person to comply with socially ascribed roles.

Religion is a central cultural instrument in the maintenance of ascribed gender roles. Religion is even worse since its followers assume that the gendered relations in their traditions, scriptures and practices are divinely sanctioned. Religions, however, are culture-specific and shaped by the culture of their origin. One typical example is the Bible. The Genesis 2-3 creation story says a man (Adam) was created first, while the woman was created from a man and for a man. Moreover, Eve's leadership, wisdom and decision-making is flawed and easily falls into a temptation, leading the whole world to disaster. Thus she is tricked by the serpent. God punishes the man saying, "Because you listened to your wife...," a statement that implies that men should not listen to their wives. Well, they can listen to their wives, just as Adam did, but at their own risk! In the story, a woman's subjugation to her husband and her mothering roles are cast as results of God's punishment. Genesis 2-3 is a master piece in the construction of gender relations that subjugates a woman to a man at multiple levels. There will be numerous other religious traditions and scriptures that propound ideologies of gender inequalities. The issue, however, is that once it is in the scripture some people say it is God's will. "God said, "You will desire your husband and she will rule over you!" In many churches, mosques and synagogues gender inequalities are often presented as God's will for the believers.

This plotting of the construction and maintenance of gender serves to underline that culture is a central instrument in the social construction of men and women. It constructs gender and maintains gender roles through various institutions and stages of life. In this way, gender seems total. To others it seems natural, while to some it seems divine. Any suggestion to change this deeply entrenched cultural system often touches on the very central nerve of our social identities and thinking. It is often resisted. People will say, "What? How do you want us to relate?" Some feel threatened and get defensive, for if they have to confront that gender construction does not share power equally, amongst women and men, they may have to share power, or as they think, they may have to loose power.

Many African men label gender activists as raving feminists, who have been listening too much to western women. They accuse those who talk of gender as imposing and importing a problem that does not exist in Africa. "Our women," they tell us, "have never been oppressed. They have always been strong and they lead us here in Africa." Describing the response of African man to the call for gender justice, T.S. Maluleke says,

> African men have responded by (a). saying, in various ways, "our women are not like that, so it must be foreign influences' that are causing them to speak and act in this manner." And (b) by fleeing from dialogue with women by suggesting that since they are not women, they will not comment on anything to do with gender…for fear of being accused of meddling (2001:238).

Maluleke continues to say, "the first response is a thin worn out excuse, while the other is deception and bigotry of the highest order" (238). Men cannot run away anymore from social responsibility. As you might know, the 2000 slogan for HIV and AIDS Day campaign was "men can make a difference." One way of making this difference in the spread of HIV and AIDS is to interrogate gender inequalities and to seek gender justice. But it is not only men who respond defensively, when issues of gender are highlighted. Some women also get upset, for they do not wish to confront their gender powerlessness. They do not want to hear about it. Well, this is understandable; people do not like to confront their powerlessness or helplessness especially if they believe that they cannot change the situation. It is better sometimes then to bury one's head in the sand. For some women, this response highlights that they have also fully embraced the socially-ascribed roles as natural, divine and unchangeable. Unfortunately, we cannot afford these excuses any more in this day and age of HIV and AIDS.

It is important that we must assume the responsibility of making a positive difference on both HIV prevention and AIDS care. Any theologian, lecturer, FBO leader or worker, who lives in the human rights era, one who believes in democracy; one who wants to be a positive contributor in the fight against HIV and AIDS, which is turning our darkly

populated continent populated into a red fire inflamed continent of death—
must not only seek to fully understand how gender is socially and
culturally constructed; how it dis-empowers half of humanity; how it fuels
the spread of HIV and AIDS—but also seek to change gender
constructions. We must seek to reconstruct gender roles such that they
empower both men and women in our communities. We must underline
that gender roles are socially constructed and it is upon the society to be
instruments of change and transformation. The present set up, does not
benefit any one—both men and women, the boys and girls of Botswana
are kissing the grave of death due to the fact that gender inequalities are a
major driving force behind the spread of HIV and AIDS.   And since
gender inequalities work together with social, cultural, economic and
political inequalities, it pervades all our lives.

Let us return to the national slogan *"Ntwa e bolotse"* (we are in a war
against HIV). Now that we know that gender inequalities are a major
driving force in the spread of HIV, are we ready to be effective soldiers in
the army? Are we ready to shoot away gender inequalities from our
relationships and society as part of arresting HIV spread from our midst? I
believe that theologians and Faith-based-leaders can and should make a
difference in building and promoting gender justice, since they train and
teach people about faith and healthy relationships, willed by God.
Relationships that promote ill-health and death are not consistent with
God's will, who is the author and creator of all life. Now, more than ever,
we need to fully understand gender roles—how they are socially
constructed and how they can be reconstructed and transformed to
empower us as men and women, as boys and girls, as elderly men and
women, as wives and husbands, as communities and nations—as people of
the black continent (Africa).   We need to reconstruct our relations so that
they do not serve as death pathways, but become life-affirming relations,
that resist poverty, powerlessness and HIV and AIDS.

Transforming Oppressive Gender Constructions through Culture

How can we transform our cultures and build gender justice within our
communities? The joy of any culture is that it is never absolute. Some
pores and windows of difference always exist. As agents of change, we
need to find these and employ them for the creation of a better world; a
just and healthy world. I would like to divide these windows of hope into
three categories. First, things that have always been within our cultures—
that contrary to gender dis-empowerment, have always insisted on a better

and more just world for all. Second, we can capitalize on a strong base of human rights culture that authorizes us to insist on the rights of all people regardless of their being black, women, young, poor, or their beliefs. To begin with the first, what are the cultural resources of our societies that empower both men and women? I am sure that as you were reading you may have said, "But but…" recalling some cultural aspects that empower both genders. We need to bring these up and find ways of using them frequently as a strategy for transformation. More often than not, these traditions are way too few and overwhelmed by the pervasiveness of gendered relations, which are well guarded in most of our crucial social institutions as well as beliefs. However, we can make it a point to strategically use the institutional spaces that we occupy in theological colleges and faith-based institutions to encourage the liberating traditions and make them more influential in the relationships of communities that we lead.

One such window of hope is from Setswana language and Bantu cultures as a whole, which are gender-neutral. We will briefly look at Setswana language on the divine department. In Setswana, *Modimo* (God) is neither given female or male names or attributes. *Mwari* of the Shona, *Nkulunkulu* of Ndebele is neither male nor female or given any gendered attributes (save with the influence of Christianity that has popularized God as, *rara,* Father). Moreover, human intermediaries such as *ngaka* (indigenous doctor), *sangoma* (spirit medium), *wosana* (rain dancer spirit medium) can be both female and male. The Setswana creation myth also features men and women coming out of the cave with their livestock. Notably, there is no hierarchy in the Setswana creation myth, nor is there a divorce of property from one gender in the story. Other powerful resources are in Setswana folk tales, the stories that teach children's moral values that, while they feature human characters, tend to feature animal characters. The impact of male-gendered characters in identity making stories has been widely studied. The Setswana animal-featuring folktales are somewhat a more gender-neutral way of socializing both genders. The animal-featuring stories can be used to critique books that constantly feature their lead characters or protagonist as males.

The above discussion of *bogwera* and *bojale* highlights that the economic gendering was that of family production: men as cattle keepers and women as crop producers—than a strictly men as bread winners of the family. The economic set up underlines that in Setswana thinking, economic or career development was never solely a male avenue. I am sure that many readers will know many of other counter- traditions that empower both genders to be public leaders, property owners and decision makers. In our *ntwa e bolotse* war against the invasion of HIV, these gender-justice promoting traditions are the bullets that we need to shoot down the HIV goliath invasion. The point, however, is that we need to find a space to use these as a counterculture strategy that subverts gender injustice and gives us the space to advocate gender justice.

Second, we are probably some of the luckiest human beings to live in the human rights century. Many centuries have passed where people were discriminated against on the grounds of their race, ethnicity, religion, age, class, physical challenge, sexual orientation and gender and they had nowhere to turn to. Many cultures sanctioned suppression of people on the basis of difference and nothing protected them. Many people lost their lives; many were persecuted because they came from ethnic groups that were despised as inferior; some because they were regarded as black, hence denied their full human rights; some because they were born with some physical challenge; some were denied their human rights just because they were born women; some have been hit hard at school for writing and eating with a left hand; twins were killed as bad omens in some cultures, some were seen and treated as dogs due to their class and age. Hey, all of us know that these things are still happening in this world and age, but no longer without a serious objection from a human rights framework perspective and the international community.

A major advantage for us today, as compared to some ancient communities, therefore, is that the international community has created a forum and created instruments that try to cultivate Human Rights-based cultures for all. Hence today we have The Human Rights charter, the Children's Charter and the Convention for the Elimination of all Forms of Discrimination Against Women, to mention just a few. Most of our governments ratified these instruments—hence giving us a mandate to use them to fight against all forms of discrimination and to cultivate values that are informed by Human Rights. In addition, The Organization of African Unity has come up with its own charters. All these are instruments of cultural change, for culture is not stagnant. It is dynamic. In sum, human rights point us to different ways of relating, where no one needs to be discriminated on the basis of their difference.

I believe in the Faith sector's commitment to life, for all life is sacred to God. The question, therefore, is: are we going to allow millions of people to die today, when we are knowingly aware that "gender inequalities are a major driving force behind the AIDS epidemic?" Gender oppressions are violations of human rights, many of which our countries have ratified. Or are we, as those who heed the call, *ntwa e bolotse,* as soldiers in the army, willing to do what it takes to establish gender justice, and significantly deprive HIV of its sting? It is up to us as religion/theologians and FBOs leaders to cultivate a gender sensitive cultures that respect the rights of all. I am confident that as believers, you harbor no conflict against the notion of Human Rights, for it is within your faith that every human being was created in God's image and deserves to live a dignified life.

The last resource that I wish to highlight is your very selves. Most social change triggers do not occur unless somebody somewhere is willing to take a stand. Gender justice requires committed people, who fully understand its dynamics and how it contributes to the spread of HIV. It needs people who are willing to pronounce the current gender constructions as unjust, unhealthy, unprofitable and to advocate for gender justice. I suggest that we must begin by examining ourselves and the programs of our theological and FBO institutions: are they gender sensitive? In short, are we gender sensitive or do we still operate within the culture of gender inequality, hence maintain the status quo? What about our homes and the relations we hold there? I suspect that most of us work within the culture of gender injustice. But I want to believe that we hold positions of responsibility in the society, as leaders, teachers, trainers or church ministers and we are partners in the search for healing. Our leadership is central in the fight against HIV and AIDS. I urge you to take your place in the front line and fight to reduce and finally eradicate the spread of HIV from our individual and social bodies. To be effective soldiers, we need to highlight how HIV and AIDS work with gender inequalities as well as to work for the establishment of gender justice. This move will have a significant impact on the prevention of HIV and AIDS given that "gender inequalities overlap with other social, cultural, economic and inequalities—and affect women and men of all ages." One strike at gender inequalities will have multiple fruits of justice in other social areas. The clarion call to do battle against HIV and AIDS has long been sounded: *ntwa e boletse!*

Bibliography

Adam, A. K. M. *Handbook of Postmodern Biblical Interpretation,* St Louis: Chalice Press, 2000.

—. *Postmodern Interpretations of the Bible, A Reader,* St Louis: Chalice Press, 2001.

Blodget, B. "Religion," Russell, L. M. and Shannon Clarkson, J. (Eds.), *Dictionary of Feminist Theologies*. Louisville: Westminster Press, 1995, 240.

Boer, R. "Culture, Ethics and Identity in Reading Ruth: A Response to Donaldson, Dube, Mackinlay and Brenner," In Brenner, A. (Ed). *A Feminist Companion to the Bible,* Sheffield: Sheffield Academic Press, 1999, 161-170

Botswana Police. Study *of Rape in Botswana.* Gaborone: Ministry of the State of the President, 1999.

Dube, M. W. (Ed.) *Other Ways of Reading, African Women and the Bible.* Atlanta: SBL, 2001.

—. "Preaching to the Converted, Unsettling the Christian Church." In *Ministerial Formation,* Vol. 93, 2000, 38-50.

—. "Grant Me Justice, Female and Male Equality in the New Testament," *Journal of Religion and Theology in Namibia*, Vol. 3, 2001, 82-115.

Childers, J. and Hentzi, G. (Eds.) *Columbia Dictionary of Modern Literary and Cultural Criticism,* New York: Colombia University Press, 1995.

Fabella, V. and Sugitharajah, R.S. (Eds.) *Dictionary of Third World Theologies.* New York: Orbis, 2000.

Gupta, G. R. "Gender, Sexuality and HIV/AIDS, The What, the Why and the How." Plenary Address XIIIth International AIDS Conference, Durban, South Africa, www.icrw.org, 2000, 1-8.

IPS. "Rights for Women Can Stem HIV/AIDS," *IPS Magazine on Gender and Human Rights*, New York: UN Special Session, 2002.

Kanyoro, M. K. "Culture," In Fabella V. and Sugirtharajah, R.S. (Eds.) *Dictionary of Third World Theologies.* New York: Orbis, 2000, 62-63.

Maluleke, T. S. "African "Ruths," Ruthless Africa's: Reflections of an African Mordecai." In Dube, M. W. (ed.), *Other Ways of Reading: African Women and the Bible,* Atlanta: Geneva: SBL/WCC, 2001, 237-251.

NACA. *The Botswana AIDS Impact Surveys III.* Gaborone: NACA, 2008.

—. *The Botswana AIDS Impact Surveys III.* Gaborone: NACA, 2004.

—. *Botswana National Strategic Framework 2003-2009,* Gaborone: Pyramid Publishing, 2003.

Oduyoye, M. A..*Daughters of Anowa: African Women and Patriarchy,* New York: Orbis, 1995.

—. *Hearing and Knowing: Theological Reflections in Africa.* New York: Orbis, 1986.

Purvis, S. "Compassion," In Russell, L. and Clarkson, S. (Eds.), *Dictionary of Feminist Theologies.* Louisville: John Knox Press, 1996, 51-52.

Schapera, I. .*A Handbook of Tswana Law and Custom,* London: Frank Cass, 1938.

Shaibu, S. and Dube.M. W. "Key Gender Issues in HIV/AIDS Prevention and Care: Towards a Gender-sensitive Multi-sectoral Approach," Gaborone: UNDP, 2002.

Soyinka, W. *The Lion and the Jewel,* London: Oxford University Press, 1963.

Surin, K. "Culture/Cultural Criticism," In Adam, A.K.M. (ed.), *Handbook for Postmodern Biblical Interpretation.* St Louis, Chalice Press, 2000, 49-54.

Tolbert, M. A. "Gender," Adam, A.K.M. (ed.), *Handbook of Postmodern Biblical Interpretation.* St Louis: Chalice Press, 2000, 99-105.

UNAIDS. *Men and AIDS, A Gendered Approach-2000 World AIDS Approach.* Geneva: UNAIDS, 2000.

—. *2008 Report on Global AIDS Epidemic,* Geneva: UNAIDS, 2008.

—. *Report on the Global HIV/AIDS Epidemic,* Geneva: UNAIDS, 2002.

UNAIDS and UNDP, *Fact Sheet, Global Crisis Global Action.* New York: United Nations Special Session On HIV/AIDS, 25-27 June, 2001.

UNDP and Botswana Government, *The Botswana Human Development Report 2000: Towards an AIDS-Free Generation.* Gaborone: UNDP, 2000.

WCC, *Making Connections, Facing Aids.* Geneva: WCC, 1993.

—. *Facing AIDS, The Challenge, the Churches' Response.* Geneva: WCC, 1997.

Wren, B. *What Language Shall I Borrow: God Talk in Worship A Male Response to Feminist Theology.* London: SCM Press, 1989.

Zizek, S. *Mapping Ideology.* London: Verso, 1994.

CHAPTER TWELVE

THE MISSING LINK:
MINORITY LANGUAGES OF BOTSWANA
IN THE FIGHT AGAINST HIV AND AIDS

JOYCE T. MATHANGWANE

Introduction

This chapter argues for the need to use other indigenous languages of Botswana in the fight against HIV and AIDS. The chapter is of the view that these languages are the missing link which could allow HIV and AIDS information to effectively reach out to speakers of these languages. Different other social fields are suggested where these other languages could be utilized to reach out, given the multi-lingual and multi-ethnic set-up of the country other than using two languages only, Setswana and English. In this regard, the paper is of the view that even where people use a second or third language, there are certain semantic values that only a first language makes the hearer or reader relate to the message and own it personally.

The chapter is based on selected AIDS messages from billboards, clinic notice boards and newspapers that were collected over a period of several years within the country. These messages were written in two languages, Setswana and English. The latest and most recent of these messages have been appearing in the newspapers and billboards. These are based on Setswana sayings and proverbs unlike the old messages. These messages are also written in both Setswana and English and under each there would be a caption educating readers on some aspect of HIV and AIDS. The chapter opens with the language situation in Botswana. This is followed by the background to HIV and AIDS epidemic in Botswana; the media and language use; the role of churches in the use of indigenous languages; NGOs, associations and language use; and, traditional healers and language use. The last section is the conclusion to the chapter.

Language situation in Botswana

Botswana, like many African countries, is both a multi-ethnic and multi-lingual country with well over 20 languages spoken within its borders (Nyati-Ramahobo (1999), Batibo, Mathangwane & Tsonope (2003), Mooko (2006), among others). These languages divide into 3 groups according to their linguistic affiliation. The majority group belongs to the Bantu family. This group comprises Setswana, Ikalanga, Sesubiya, Thimbukushu, Shiyeyi, Otjiherero, Shekgalagarhi, Sebirwa, and Setswapong and a few others such as Silozi, IsiNdebele spoken by comparatively fewer speakers in the country. As noted by Mathangwane (2002) among others, this group makes up over 96 per cent of the population. The second group of languages belongs to the Khoesan family which makes up about 3 per cent of the population. Even though this group is relatively small, it comprises a large number of languages used in Botswana such as Ju/'hoan, Naro, !Xoo, /Xaise, Danisi, Nama, //Gana, Cara, Tshwa, Kua, /Gwi, Sasi, Hietshware, Ts'ixa, /Anda, Kxoe, Deti, Buga, Shuakwe, ǂKx'au/'ein, ǂHua and other small groups. The third group is that of the Indo-European family which in Botswana consists almost entirely of Afrikaans spoken mainly in the Tsabong and Gantsi areas in the western parts of the country. It constitutes a very small number of about 0.2 per cent of the population. English though widely used in the country, is largely as a second language.

Of the languages spoken in the country, Setswana is the majority language spoken by a high percentage of the population. Andersson and Janson (1997) estimate 70% to 90%; Nyati-Ramahobo (1999) estimates 80%; Batibo (2005) estimates 78.6%, etc. English and Setswana enjoy some recognition in the sense that both are used in the education system and administrative circles while the rest are relegated to use in their own communities. English is the official language of the country and is the medium of instruction from standard two up to tertiary level, while Setswana, is the medium of instruction at standard one in the primary schools. All the other languages in the country tend to be marginalized and are with no official status within the country. As a result, there has been little or no development of these other languages in terms of orthographies or reading and teaching materials. This is even more so with the Khoesan languages, which are the most vulnerable because of the history of domination of their speakers by other groups. As pointed out by Mooko (2006), among others, such a situation as we have in the country is a threat to other indigenous languages. Even in more danger than others are some

Khoesan languages which are no longer spoken by the younger generation in their communities.

However, in the past ten years or so, orthographies of some of these other languages have been developed or are in the process of being developed. Those with developed orthographies include Shiyeyi, Nama, Naro, Ikalanga, Ju/'hoan, Afrikaans, Otjiherero, Isindebele, Silozi, Thimbukushu, Nambya, Shekgalagarhi, and Zezuru, while those which are still being developed include Chikuhane/Sesubiya, Sebirwa, Khwedam, !Xoo, and Rugciriku. For some of these languages, the orthographies exist in the neighboring countries where these languages are also used. Languages without orthographies are not included here.

Background to HIV and AIDS Epidemic in Botswana

The first case of HIV and AIDS in Botswana was identified in 1985 and it is estimated that significant spread of HIV in the country started in the mid 1980's. Since then, the spread of the virus in the population has been explosive. With this outbreak, the government of Botswana introduced some strategies to fight against the pandemic. One such strategy was by launching a widespread and intensive campaign to educate people on how to avoid HIV. This campaign included disseminating messages that speak of the dire consequences of AIDS and of the need to avoid contracting HIV. To-date such messages are all over the country. Beginning 2008 new messages based on Setswana sayings appear in the weekly local newspapers and some billboards. In addition to these, other messages appear on Botswana Television (Btv) as sketches. These messages though, are in two languages only, that is, Setswana and English. This is irrespective of the fact that Botswana is a multi-lingual and multi-ethnic country. The billboard messages are found throughout the country even in those rural areas where most speakers are not mother tongue speakers of Setswana. The assumption has always been that the majority of Batswana can speak, understand and read in Setswana. However, this is not always the case, especially with the older generations in the non-Setswana speaking groups. In the year 2000, the National AIDS Coordinating Agency (NACA) was launched through which His Excellency the then President of Botswana, Mr Festus Mogae, declared war against HIV/AIDS. In addition, government has made available Anti-Retroviral (ARV) treatment to those already infected in partnership with the African Comprehensive HIV and AIDS Partnerships (ACHAP), among others. These partnerships are committed to provide more assistance to Botswana until 2009 in its fight against the scourge. In order to further demonstrate its commitment to the fight against this pandemic, the government came up with The National HIV and AIDS Strategic Framework 2003 – 2009 whose main goal was "to eliminate the incidence of HIV and reduce the impact of AIDS in Botswana".   This is a clear indication that the government of Botswana together with its partners is committed to fight this scourge. Given the magnitude of this scourge, it is critical that all resources available be used and that includes the use of other indigenous languages in the country.

In his statement at a Panel Discussion on "Breaking the Cycle of HIV Infection for Sustainable AIDS Responses" held in New York on the 31st May 2006, His Excellency the former President of Botswana Mr Festus Mogae observed that some of the dimensions which affect the rate of HIV/AIDS infection "… suggest the influence of deeply rooted factors such as culture and tradition" (Tautona Times No.18 of 2006 – The Weekly Electronic Press Circular of the Office of the President). Thus, to effectively address a multidimensional problem such as HIV and AIDS, requires that government takes cognizance of the people's culture and traditions which calls for government communicating with the people through the medium of their own languages because it is in the people's language that their moral values, norms and taboos about sex and sexuality are conveyed from one generation to the next.

The media and language use

As noted in Mathangwane & Smieja (2000), mass media in Botswana date as far back as the mid 1800's with publications such as Molokai we Batswana (1856-1857), Northern News (1914) Lesedi la Batswana (about 1930) Kutlwano (1963) to mention a few. To-date media in Botswana has really grown. Not only has there been an increase in the number of newspapers produced locally, the number of local radio stations has also increased. There are altogether five radio stations, that is, RB1, RB2, YaRona FM, GABZ FM and the recently launched DUMA FM. The only glitch is that not all these stations are accessed in all parts of the country. So far only two of these radio stations are accessible throughout the country and these are RB1 and RB2. However, recently there has been a move to spread accessibility of other stations such as GABZ FM to other parts of the country. In addition, there are several local newspapers whose circulation reaches most of the major villages, towns and cities of the country. Botswana Television (Btv) which came into being in 2000 is accessible throughout the country if one has a satellite dish. Despite this growth, one major setback in the media is that communication is mainly in

English and Setswana. Up to about 2007 or so, one could come across an article written in Ikalanga in the Mmegi newspaper, which practice seems to have stopped.

The recent move by NACA and its partners to place AIDS messages in the weekly newspapers and billboards targeting couples (married or unmarried) based on Setswana proverbs is a step in the right direction, though on billboards along the roads, the messages are too detailed to read for drivers while driving. These messages are given in Setswana and English and under each proverb/saying is a message cautioning against such behavior and the consequences on the spread of HIV. Below are examples of such messages.

(a)   Message A (Setswana):
        "Batho bare ... 'Monna gaa botswe otswa kae'
        Mme go ikgatholosa dilo tse gogo baya mo diphatseng tsago tsenwa ke
        mogare wa HIV.
        Mogare wa HIV o anama motlhofo mo dibekeng tsa ntlha morago ga go tsenwa ke mogare, pele ga motho aka itse gore o tsenwe ke mogare. Jaanong fa o sa botse ka metsamao ya mokapelo wa gago, ga o itse gore a o go baya mo diphatseng tsa go tsenwa ke mogare wa HIV." (translation: 'HIV is easily transmitted in the first weeks after infection by the virus before a person is aware of the infection. If you do not ask about your partner's sexual behaviors, you never know if you are in danger of HIV infection'.)

(b)   Message B (English):
        "A Setswana saying goes ... 'Never asks a man about his comings and goings'
        But turning a blind eye puts you at risk of HIV.
        The more often you have sex with someone who is HIV positive, the more likely you will become HIV positive yourself. And HIV spreads most easily in the first few weeks after infection, before a person even knows they are infected. So if you don't ask about your partner's coming and goings, you don't know if he is putting you at risk of HIV."

(c)   Message C (Setswana):
        "Batho ba re ... 'Monna ga a agelwe legora'.
        Mme o ka anamisa mogare go tswa mo legoreng le lengwe go yak o go le lengwe.

Mogare wa HIV o anama motlhofo mo dibekeng tsa ntlha morago ga go tsenwa ke mogare wa HIV, pele le ha motho a ka itse gore o tsenwe ke mogare. Ka jalo, fa monna a ka se agelwe legora o itsenya mmogo le mokapelo wa gagwe mo diphatseng tsa go tsenwa ke mogare was HIV." (translation: And HIV spreads most easily in the first few weeks after infection, before a person even knows they are infected. So, when a man cannot be contained in one kraal he is putting himself and his partner at risk of HIV".

(d)   Message D (English):
"A Setswana saying goes ... 'A man can't be contained in one kraal'. But he can spread HIV from one kraal to another.
The more often you have sex with someone who is HIV positive, the more likely you will become HIV positive yourself. And HIV spreads most easily in the first few weeks after infection, before a person even knows they are infected. So, when a man cannot be contained in one kraal he is putting himself and his partner at risk of HIV".

In their study, Chilisa, Bennell and Hyde (2001) noted that about two thirds of the students in the focus group discussions they conducted agreed with the statement that 'cultural beliefs expose women to the risk of contracting HIV/AIDS'. As a result, young women are said to be further exposed to the risk of HIV/AIDS because such cultural beliefs and practices encourage men to have multiple partners. Such beliefs are generally reflected in sayings/proverbs such as have been used in these latest NACA messages. Chilisa, Bennell and Hyde (2001:17) cite the following as some of the common sayings which have been passed from generation to generation:

"Monna ke poo ga a agelelwe losaka (A man is a bull to be let loose)
Monna ke thotse oa nama (A man is a seed to multiply)
Monna ke selepe oa adimanwa (A man is an axe to be exchanged)."

The fact that these HIV messages respond to these sayings pointing out the dire consequences of such behavior are invaluable lessons against some of these cultural beliefs. The missing link in this case is not using such sayings/proverbs in the other indigenous languages of Botswana to educate mother tongue speakers. Proverbs, as noted in Yusuf and Mathangwane (2003), among others, can be a very useful tool to provide deep understanding of the magnitude of the HIV problem as they are steeped in the traditions and cultures of the people. Thus, NACA should consider using such sayings/proverbs from other local languages also to reach out to these other communities. Such messages would prove most helpful as they would reflect and draw from the cultural beliefs of the people.

Many studies have shown that the media is a very strong tool when reaching out to communities or educating them on some important aspects of their lives. It is a very powerful tool which can direct and set an agenda on issues of importance. This is a fact known to politicians in Botswana as well as the world over. For instance, in the period leading to the 2004 elections, Botswana Television (Btv) broadcasted messages urging people to go and vote using other indigenous languages. Such languages included Ikalanga, Otjiherero, Shekgalagarhi, and Afrikaans. These messages were highly thought of and speakers of these languages were enchanted to see their languages spoken on television. For many, it raised a sense of pride to hear these messages in their languages. Even though a small number of Botswana languages was used, this is an important indication that the decision makers are aware of the importance of communicating with people in the languages that they understand and own. Another example is that of BOTUSA (Botswana – USA Partnership) an organization doing research on HIV and AIDS in the country. In the Francistown area in the northern part of Botswana where a dominant number of residents are Ikalanga speakers, in addition to Setswana, some of their consent forms are written in Ikalanga and in homes which are Ikalanga speaking, these are the consent forms used because it is important that people give their consent in a language of their own which they understand very well (Mathangwane 2009). HIV messages should also be tailor-made in different ethnic languages other than Setswana and English only if Botswana were to eradicate this pandemic.

In their study on future trends in the media, Mathangwane and Smieja (2000) observed that a significant percentage of respondents prefer that other ethnic languages of Botswana be used on radio and television. The use of these languages would not only enrich the cultural diversity of the country but will also bring about better understanding through effective communication especially in the areas of health, agriculture, and politics, among others. This is in spite of some stereotypes among other people that other indigenous languages are difficult to read or write. Such stereotypes are definitely a legacy of the education system of the country where only two languages Setswana and English are being used to the detriment of all the others. There is no language that is difficult to read or write. It is people's habits that make it difficult to adjust to written and spoken forms of other languages.

The Role of the Churches in the use of indigenous languages

The good work of Churches in Botswana in the promotion and development of other indigenous languages is above reproach. A good example is the work of Hessel and Coby Visser among the Naro in D'Kar, Gantsi District under the auspices of the Church Council of the Reformed Church in Botswana. Working together with the Kuru Development Trust (a trust set up by the Reformed Church in Botswana), not only have they achieved high standards in developing the Naro language, but have also given hope for the future to the Naro people by working towards creating jobs and fighting such social ills as alcoholism (Visser 2000). The Vissers are said to have also developed materials on the fight against the HIV and AIDS pandemic. Also worth mentioning are the works of the Lutheran Church in promoting local languages such as Ikalanga, !Xoon, Shekgalagarhi, among others, through the likes of Rev. Richard Cook who was based at Thamaga, Rev. Daniel Schmitt in Francistown, and Rev. David Lang at Okwi village in the Kgalagadi north.

The role of Churches should not be underestimated because their influence in the communities they serve is very crucial. The fact that the Christian messages minister to the souls of congregants means that whoever uses a language of the soul will touch many and bring them to comply with the requirements of the message. Even politicians in the western countries are known to work hard to win the support of the Christian coalitions in order to win elections.

However, in the fight against the HIV and AIDS scourge, Churches in Botswana should have taken a more active role to address people in their own ethnic languages in those areas where these languages are dominant, especially when praying for those that are sick or dying from HIV and AIDS; or, when counseling and educating people about HIV and AIDS. Prayers, counseling and even lessons delivered in one's own language are more highly appreciated by mother tongue speakers. Also, to use one's language is to observe the culture of that person which may not be understood or appreciated by an outsider. The problem has always been the assumption that everyone in the country speaks and understands Setswana, which is not always the case. Churches ought to preach and deliver messages against HIV in other indigenous languages within their own cultural contexts. As a result, people would feel ownership and appreciation bringing about the desired behavior change. Understandably so, some languages do not as yet have the Bible translation or hymn books. In such cases, translators could be used in order to reach out to the communities. The same applies to social gatherings such as funerals where there are people from different ethnic groups. Rather than using Setswana, as seems to be the practice, other local languages should also be used. The importance of Churches in influencing language practices is further noted in Nyati-Ramahobo (1999:93) as she writes:

> Church is a social domain in which language use can be observed due to the organized nature of the proceedings. The church can also be very influential domain in the implementation of a language policy in the sense that the language used in the church reaches large audiences hence its spread. Language of the church is also associated with sacredness and holiness and it is respected. Churches make their own literature and therefore, contribute to the implementation of the language policy.

NGOs, Associations, Cultural Groups and language use

There are several NGOs (Non-Government Organizations), associations and cultural groups in Botswana which have been working towards saving some of the indigenous languages. Most of these are formations by speakers of these indigenous languages in their quest to save their languages, and their primary objective is to promote and preserve these languages and the culture of the people. Some of the associations have been in existence for more than a decade now, while others may be quite recent. Likewise their achievements vary depending on how active they have been and the length of time they have been in existence. The table below provides a list of these associations and cultural groups and the languages they are working to promote.

Table 1: NGO's, Associations and Cultural Groups working on other indigenous languages

Name of Associations	Languages
Society for Promotion of Ikalanga Language (SPIL) Mukani Action Campaign	Ikalanga
Kamanakao Association	Shiyeyi
Qonyathe Cnsha	!Xoo
Teemashane Community Trust Trust for Okavango Cultural and Development Initiatives (TOCaDI)	Khwedam
Mbungu wa ka Thimana The Language Learning Centre at Etsha	Thimbukushu
Chelwa ya Shekgalagarhi	Shekgalagarhi
Lentswe la Batswapong Association	Setswapong
The Kuru Development Trust at D'Kar	Naro
Cisiya-Nkulu Trust	Cisubiya (Chikuhane)
The First People of the Kalahari	Basarwa Languages
Babirwa Cultural Group	Sebirwa
Baherero-Banderu Youth Club	Otjiherero

The last three in the table are cultural groups. In addition to the above which focus on individual languages, there are some that have broader aims which include WIMSA (Working Group of Indigenous Minorities of Southern Africa), assisting most of the Khoesan languages, and RETENG: The Multi-Cultural Coalition of Botswana whose primary objective is "to promote cultural diversity, multi-lingualism and social justice" in Botswana (www.reteng.org). RETENG works towards the cultural development of all the other indigenous languages of Botswana.

All the above should play a crucial role in disseminating information on HIV and AIDS in these languages and help fight the HIV pandemic. In a country wide study that was carried out by Batibo, Mathangwane and Tsonope (2003), most of the communities to which these associations and cultural groups belong responded that they would love to see their languages used in social domains. Some of these Associations and cultural groups hold annual cultural events which could prove very effective in communicating HIV and AIDS messages in the languages of the local communities. Such messages could be in the form of song, dance, poetry, plays, etc. which will be meaningful to speakers of the respective languages. The Khoesan languages which, in most cases, are used publicly in official functions when songs and dance are performed could also be utilized to disseminate the messages on HIV and AIDS in their own communities. In other words, these indigenous languages forums could effectively and inexpensively disseminate messages for combating the HIV and AIDS pandemic. For instance, the Domboshaba celebrations of the Bakalanga held annually, where materials on HIV and AIDS written in Ikalanga could be made available to Ikalanga speakers.

Traditional leaders and language use

Traditional leaders play a very important role in their communities, leading and guiding the people. Chieftainship is part of the culture of all Batswana and each ethnic group has a chief or sub-chief responsible for guiding and leading the people. Therefore, to reach out to people of all tribal groups in the country, chiefs are of paramount importance. It is the role of these leaders to educate people on matters relating to HIV and AIDS and admonish people on any unbecoming behavior which may endanger their wellbeing. *Kgotla* meetings addressed in the local languages would have a great impact reaching out to the communities.

Proverbs and other sayings in all these languages could also be put to good use at such meetings. As noted by several scholars working on proverbs, proverbs are considered to be strategies for dealing with situations (see Yusuf and Mathangwane (2003:408); Mieder & Holmes (2000:92), among others). In difficult situations people have been known to turn to proverbs for answers, and they find them. Using proverbs from Ikalanga, Yoruba and English, Yusuf and Mathangwane demonstrated that proverbs can be related to different aspects of the fight against HIV and AIDS, that is, HIV and AIDS campaign, HIV and AIDS Care-giving and living with HIV and AIDS. All the indigenous languages of Botswana are rich with proverbs which can be used to communicate and reach out to people on this scourge. Proverbs are in actual fact the best tools for conveying such messages because proverbs reflect the cultural diversity of the people. Elders in these communities could work hand in hand with the Chiefs and address their communities using appropriate language within each cultural context to convey very strong messages on the need to change behavioral attitudes in the fight against HIV. Role models too would play key roles alongside the elders and the Chiefs in order to come up with effective communication strategies suitable for the target groups and, equally important, strategies sensitive to the cultural values and practices of the communities.

It is therefore clear that language, as a vehicle for conveying the social and intellectual values and qualities of any human community, has a special role in the life of individuals. The subtle euphemisms of each language have a greater effect on speakers than plain tart messages in languages that are acquired later in life. There is ownership, attraction and pride when one hears a message in the language of one's cultural, spiritual and linguistic values.

Conclusion

This chapter set out to look at the importance of indigenous languages in the fight against HIV and AIDS in Botswana. The paper noted that the war against the HIV and AIDS is a mammoth task which the whole nation should take part and own. Thus, if we are to emerge victorious in this way, all the indigenous languages of Botswana should be used in disseminating information and messages on HIV and AIDS. In this study, several HIV messages were collected from billboards, clinics' notice boards and newspapers. All these messages are in two languages, Setswana and English. The chapter argues that the missing link in the fight against this pandemic is lack of use of the other indigenous languages of Botswana. In those areas which are dominant of other indigenous languages, the local languages would be more effective because they would reflect the culture of the people. As a result, speakers would identify with the language used bringing about the desired change in behavior. In other words, the importance of mother tongue languages should not be underestimated when trying to reach out to communities be it for pedagogy or educating society on social ills such as HIV and AIDS. The use of these other indigenous languages would facilitate officials tasked with educating people understand the cultural beliefs of other ethnic groups as a result come up with effective strategies to combat the spread of this virus throughout the nation.

The chapter further notes that the media, Churches, NGOs, associations and cultural groups and traditional leaders all have an important role to play. This collective effort can achieve its main goal by bringing in other indigenous languages in the fight against this scourge. In so doing, we will achieve our goal in educating the masses and bring about the desired behavior change. Proverbs and other sayings from these indigenous languages would be some of the most useful tools, a direction already taken by NACA in the latest messages that have been appearing in the local newspapers.

Bibliography

Andersson, L-G and T. Janson, *Languages in Botswana: Language Ecology in Southern Africa*, Gaborone: Longman Botswana, 1999.

Batibo, H.M., *Language Decline and Death in Africa: Causes, Consequences and Challenges*, Clevedon: Multilingual Matters Ltd, 2005.

Batibo, H.M., J.T. Mathangwane and J. Tsonope, *A Study of the Third Language Teaching in Botswan -. Consultancy Report*, (Republic of Botswana – Tender No.CTB 6/1/50/98-99 (re-advertisement), 2003.

Botswana National Strategic Framework for HIV/AIDS, 2003-2009.

Chilisa, B. with P. Bennell & K. Hyde, *The Impact of HIV/AIDS on the University of Botswana: Developing a Comprehensive Strategic Response*, UK: Department for International Development DFID, 2001.

Masa Antiretroviral Therapy, Vol.19: February 2006.

Mathangwane, J.T., "Language as a Tool for Conveying Messages on HIV/AIDS: the case of Botswana", in Odebunmi, A., Arua, A.E., Arimi, S. (eds.), *Language, Gender and Politics: A Festschrift for Y.K. Yusuf.* Lagos: Centre for Black and African Arts and Civilization, 2009, 574

Mathangwane, J.T., "An Attempt at Harmonisation or What: On the Development of the Orthographies of Botswana Languages", In K.K. Prah (ed). *Writing African: The Harmonisation of Orthographic Conventions in African Languages*, Cape Town: CASAS Book Series No.25, 2002, 65-87.

Mathangwane, J.T. and Birgit Smieja, "Future Trends in the Botswana Media: The Destiny of Minority Languages", In H.M. Batibo and B. Smieja (eds), *Botswana: the Future of Minority Languages.* Frankfurt am Main: Peter Lang, 2000, 105-125.

Mieder, W. & D. Holmes, *Children and Proverbs Speak the Truth: Teaching Proverbial Wisdom to Fourth Graders*, Burlington, Vermont: The University of Vermont Press, 2000.

Mooko, T., "Counteracting the Threat of Language Death: The case of Minority Languages in Botswana. In *Journal of Multilingual and Multicultural Development*, Vol.27: 2, 2006, 109 – 125.

Ntshebe, O., J.M.N. Pitso and A.K. Segobye, "The Use of Culturally Themed HIV messages and their implications for future behavior change communication campaigns: the case of Botswana", *Journal of Social Aspects of HIV/AIDS*, Vol. 3, 2006, 466-476.

Nyati-Ramahobo, L., *The National Language: a Resource or a Problem*, Gaborone: Pula Press, 1999.

RETENG website: www.reteng.org

Statement by His Excellency Mr Festus G. Mogae, President of the Republic of Botswana at a Panel Discussion of "Breaking the Cycle of HIV Infection for Sustainable Aids Responses" at New York on the 31st May 2006. Tautona Times No.18 of 2006. The Weekly Electronic Press Circular of the Office of the President.

Visser, Hessel, "Language and Cultural Empowerment of the Khoesan People: The Naro Experience", In H. Batibo and B. Smieja (eds), *Botswana: The Future of the Minority Languages*. Frankfurt am Main: Peter Lang, 2000, 193-215.

Yusuf, Y.K. and Joyce T. Mathangwane "Proverbs and HIV/AIDS", In *Proverbium: Yearbook of International Proverb Scholarship*, Vol.20. Vermont: The University of Vermont Press, 2003, 407-422.

Contributors

James N. Amanze is an Associate Professor of Systematic Theology and Christian Ethics at the University of Botswana. He has published widely in referred journals and books. He has also edited several books with his latest being *Christian Ethics and HIV/AIDS in Africa*. Amanze is also the editor of *BOLESWA: Journal of Theology, Religion and Philosophy*.

Musa W. Dube is a Professor of New Testament at the University of Botswana. Her research interests include gender, indigenous ways of reading the text, HIV&AIDS and postcolonial studies. Dube is the author of *The HIV&AIDS Bible: Selected Essays* and the editor of *Other Ways of Reading: African Women and the Bible*. She has received several international awards on her work on HIV and AIDS, the Bible and the church.

Joseph B.R. Gaie is a Senior Lecturer in Philosophy at the University of Botswana and current Head of Department of Theology and Religious Studies. He is a Fogarty fellow of the Berman Institute of Bioethics, Johns Hopkins University (USA) (2010 Post-Doctoral Fellowship) and a volunteer ethics teacher for pre-major seminary students and novices as well as a catechists. His research is focused on the application of ethics to different issues such as HIV, business and education. He has published widely in these areas. He is also exploring ways in which the Setswana concept of Botho can be integrated into the philosophical discourse. To this end he co-edited the book, *The Setswana Concept of HIV/AIDS in Botswana* by Zapf Chancery (2007). He had earlier published *The Ethics of Medical Involvement in Capital Punishment: A Philosophical Discussion* in 2004 by Kluwer Academic Publishers. Dr Gaie indigenizes philosophy and sees himself as a Kantian with Utilitarian inclinations.

Muhammed Haron studied at the Durban-Westville, Riyadh, Cape Town, South Africa, the Vrije Universiteit te Amsterdam and Rhodes. He taught at the Universities of Western Cape and Cape Town and is Associate Professor in Religious Studies at the University of Botswana. He was visiting lecturer at National University of Malaysia, Stellenbosch and Rhodes. He compiled *South Africa's Truth and Reconciliation Commission (circa 1993-2008): An Annotated Bibliography* (NY: Nova Science 2009) and *Muslims in South Africa: An Annotated Bibliography* (Cape Town: South African Library 1997), edited *Going Forward: South Africa-Malaysia Relations Cementing South-South Connections* (KL: Lim Kok Wing University 2008), authored *The Dynamics of Christian-Muslim Relations in South Africa (ca 1960-2000)* (Uppsala: Alqmvist 2006), and he co-authored *First Steps* and *Second Steps in Arabic Grammar* (Chicago: Iqra International Publishers 2007 & 2009).

Kipton E. Jensen (PhD, Marquette University, USA, 1996) taught philosophy at the University of Botswana between 2004 and 2008. Jensen has published on the importance of African Communalism to the design of public health programs (African Journal of AIDS Research), the ethics of HIV testing policies (WHO Policy & Practice), and religious identity in Botswana (African Identities). He presently teaches philosophy at Morehouse College in Atlanta, Georgia.

Leila Katirayi is research associate at the Elizabeth Glaser Pediatric AIDS Foundation (EGPAF) in Washington D.C. Ms. Katirayi works with the staff in EGPAF's country offices to design and implement operations research to strengthen the uptake of PMTCT and ART services in southern, eastern and western Africa. Most recently she was involved in the design and implementation of a large operations research training to build staff capacity in the country offices. Her interests are in behavioral research focused around HIV/AIDS issues. Ms. Katirayi received her undergraduate degrees at the University of Washington and her M.S. in International Development and Management at Lund University in Sweden.

Obed N. Kealotswe is a Senior Lecturer in Systematic Theology and African Independent Churches at the University of Botswana. Kealotswe has vast experience researching and writing on African Independent Churches in Botswana. He has published several articles in referred journals and several chapters in books. He recently (2007) edited *Christian*

Ethics and HIV/AIDS in Botswana with James Amanze and Fidelis Nkomazana.

Joyce T. Mathangwane is an Associate Professor of Language and Linguistics in the Department of English, University of Botswana. She has published widely in the areas of phonology and morphology of Bantu languages, sociolinguistics, comparative linguistics, onomastics and the social aspects of HIV and AIDS.

Sana K. Mmolai is a lecturer in the Department of Languages and Social Sciences Education, University of Botswana. Dr Mmolai obtained her first degree and her Post Graduate Diploma in Education from the University of Botswana. She obtained her Masters and PhD degrees from Lancaster University, majoring in Religious Education. She has taught for more than 20 years at the University of Botswana. She has participated in numerous workshops, seminars, conferences and projects on HIV/AIDS in Botswana. Her areas of interest include: the role of Religious Education in the fight against HIV/AIDS in Botswana, Faith Based Organizations' HIV Prevention Strategies; and Religious Education and the promotion of Botswana's Vision 2016. She is involved in a number of community development activities.

Fidelis Nkomazana is Senior Lecturer in church history in the Department of Theology and Religious Studies at the University of Botswana. He trained as a church historian at the University of Edinburgh, where he received his Master of Theology and PhD in 1990 and 1994 respectively. He is widely researched and published on church history and other related aspects. He is currently working on the histories of the Anglican Church, Roman Catholic Church, Pentecostalism, and Dutch Reformed Church in Botswana. He has published several books on Religious and Moral Education in secondary schools. His other research works are on the traditional religion, the role of women in the history of the church in Botswana, religion and HIV and AIDS and ecumenical movements. He has served as the Faculty Tutor for the Faculty of Humanities for more than five years and also as Head of the Department of Theology and Religious Studies at the University of Botswana for six and half years. From 2001 to 2002 he spent his twelve months Sabbatical Leave at Fuller Seminary in Pasadena, California.

Lovemore Togarasei teaches Biblical Studies and is Associate Professor in the Department of Theology and Religious Studies, University of Botswana. He takes interest in research in the areas of the Bible in African Christianity with special reference to the New Testament, Pentecostal expressions of Christianity in Africa and the public role of the church in Africa. He has led several research projects and consultancies in the area of church and public health especially HIV and AIDS. This book is a product of one of the research projects he has led. He recently (2010) edited *Faith in the City: The role and place of religion in Harare* with Ezra Chitando.